To my wife
Caroline L. Simpson

DATE DUE

Contents

Introduction

On a somnolent June afternoon, during the peaceful but ominous interbellum period of somewhat more than forty years ago, a colonel in the medical corps of the United States Army was conducting a handful of medical students on a tour of Fort Devens in mid-Massachusetts. The entire area was a mere skeleton in equipment, buildings, and manpower. The embers of the first world conflagration, for which the installation had been constructed, had long since died away and most of the huge reservation had grown up to weeds and grass while dozens of wooden barracks had fallen into decay. None of us—for I was one of the medical students—could yet hear the tramp of thousands of feet that in a few years would again shake the very ground where we now walked, slightly bored, slightly amused.

The colonel who was conducting us on our tour was a medical and military professional in every sense of the word and pointed out various sanitary needs and problems as we went along. Finally, more or less by chance, we wandered into an abandoned ruin of a warehouse. I doubt if a soul had entered the structure in a decade. For the most part, except for a scattering of litter, the building was empty, but as one door was opened we suddenly saw piled at one end of a room, actually from floor to ceiling, an enormous number of toilet seats. The sight was so unexpected for these very sophisticated medical students and so utterly ridiculous that we began to laugh. But the old colonel as he stood there viewing the scene and his callow companions murmured, "It takes a hell of a lot of things besides guns to fight a war."

ix

In the same way it might be said that it takes a lot of things besides guns to conquer a wilderness, to found a nation, to establish a democracy. The history of a nation is like a great river. You can no more understand a nation by viewing the current scene than you can understand a river by viewing it from one point on the bank. To understand a river you must know its source and follow it as it gathers tributaries, passes over turbulent rapids, rushes through mountain gorges, widens out in placid terrain, shrinks with droughts and swells with rains, and, reaching its flood, sweeps on its way to its destiny, the sea. So it is with a nation. The sources of its power are many; the influences that alter its direction or change its goals may be racial, political, geographic, or military. To write the whole history of a nation would require consideration of all these factors. Obviously the matter is too complex to be so dealt with in a nation as vast as ours, so a multitude of specialized treatises has appeared covering one, or a few, of these influences on our national development. The result is shelf after library shelf of books devoted to the effect on our culture of military campaigns, diplomacy, political parties, social reform, the industrial revolution, and dozens of other motifs. Perhaps many facets in our national evolution have been neglected; certainly one has been completely ignored, namely the impact of disease on American history. True, there are medical histories dealing with America as well as the rest of the world, but medical histories, for the most part, are drab accounts of scientific discoveries, dreary biographical sketches of physicians, or descriptions of epidemics as they affected the course of medical knowledge. Not one of them concerns itself with the overall effect of disease on the history of this nation.

If the medical historians have avoided the subject, it is scarcely surprising that the general historians have done so. Who would want to write about a sick Indian when he could describe the raids of King Philip? Who would want to read about dysentery when he could thrill to the resonant oratory of Daniel Webster? Who could find drama in a measles epidemic compared to the magnificence and tragedy of Pickett's charge at Gettysburg? And yet there may be historical significance, high tragedy, and stirring drama in stories of trumpets that never sounded, or sails that were not unfurled. The victory may go to the strongest legions, but their strength may be in numbers, in fire-power, or in immunity to infection.

Nothing in the pages that follow is intended to decry the importance of military strategy, legislative decisions, or social reform on our national maturity.

The intent is merely to demonstrate that oftentimes the difference between triumph and disaster has been due to things besides heroism, leadership, or eloquence; to things besides strength, organization, or wealth; to things besides climate, geography, or resources; and that our destiny has been molded by forces unseen and unknown, by invisible powers, invisible armies.

1
Conquest of a Continent

THE BEACHHEAD

As the fifteenth century drew to a close the nations of Europe were facing up to an enormous enterprise. This was the discovery and exploration of half a world. True, the earliest explorers had no conception of the magnitude of their undertaking. None was aware that a New World lay before him rather than just another approach to the Orient. None was aware that two huge continents stood in his path. And yet, although the immensity of the task may have been entirely unrealized, it was successfully accomplished in spite of what might have been overwhelming odds.

There were many elements contributing to the ultimate success of the explorers and colonists who established and maintained a beachhead, and who finally occupied both North and South America. The first Europeans to arrive in the New World had several advantages on their side. They were accustomed to serving a central authority with the economy of action such a discipline imparts. They understood military principles—the concept of command and leadership. They had powerful motives—the urge to serve themselves, their king, or sometimes their God. Among their own national groups, whether Spanish, French, or English, there were no communication barriers. They had supremacy on the waterways because of their naval experience and their ships. Man for man they had

1

overwhelming superiority in their weapons—they had guns.

On the other hand the Europeans had several serious handicaps. They were greatly outnumbered by battling Indians who were fighting on their own ground for their own homes, and who were thoroughly familiar with the terrain. Most important of all, the whites were forced to maintain a supply line so extensive that it seems incredible that they managed to succeed in their conquest. The reason they did succeed is one that is usually overlooked. The Europeans were able to conquer America not because of their military genius, or their religious motivation, or their ambition and avarice. They conquered it by waging unpremeditated biological warfare.

When Columbus made a landfall in Hispaniola the land was bright. Those who swiftly followed him discovered and explored an abundant territory populated for the most part by a remarkably healthy race. At that time there were probably not more than two million natives in North America, and not many more than one million in what is now the United States and Canada. The indigenous population was limited more by the available food supply than by disease. Death among the Indians was commonly due to violence, accidents, exposure, flood, famine, or old age. Contagion was not a frequent hazard as evidenced by the established fact that when the Europeans arrived there was practically no natural or racial immunity to infectious disease among the natives. There is even more direct evidence. Las Casas, whose father and uncle had come to Hispaniola with Columbus on the second voyage, and who came there himself in 1500 and was to spend most of the remainder of his life in the New World, repeatedly commented on the healthful climate. He praised Hispaniola and Central America, described the Lucayan Islands as the most healthful region of the world, and called Nicaragua a veritable nursery of men.

In 1502 Columbus explored the Central American

mainland, spending several months with his crews on land or just offshore. Their accounts of this expedition contain scarcely a single mention of sickness. There are graphic descriptions of the ferocity of the natives, the luxuriance of the vegetation and the amplitude of the harbors, but nothing about fevers. Several chroniclers, including Oviedo who came to America in 1513, made careful observations regarding the climate, flora and fauna, but made no mention of malaria, yellow fever, or any other epidemic disease.

Something must have happened. These same areas were shortly to become infamous for pestilence. Wherever the whites made more than the briefest of visits, epidemics soon became rampant. When Columbus discovered Hispaniola the island had an estimated population of 300,000 natives. Within half a century the Tainos had been practically exterminated by slaughter and starvation, but especially by smallpox.

The military problem that faced Cortes in 1519 when he set out to conquer Mexico would stagger a modern tactician. The Aztecs were brave and intelligent and were fighting on their native soil. Cortes with his tiny force conquered a kingdom and established a government that endured for three centuries. Before this campaign was completed, another expedition was sent out under Panfilo de Narvaez which contained in its entourage a black man acutely ill with smallpox. This was a crucial event in the annals of New Spain. The Indians had never encountered such a disease. They had no immunity against it. The entire countryside was stricken and the mortality was all the more ghastly because the natives, in their terror of the fever and the revolting pustules on their skins, plunged into the rivers for relief and choked the waterways with their dead.

Similar events occurred in Central and South America. Spanish historians describe an epidemic, probably smallpox, occurring in Peru several years before the conquest. This was presumably introduced by earlier Spanish explorations along the coast, of which there were many. The emperor Huayna Capac and more than two hundred thousand Peruvians were swept away in a holocaust a few years before the major assault by the Spanish. This devastation simplified the logistics and hastened the success of Pizarro's merciless destruction of the Incan empire.

Epidemics were not limited to the areas under Spanish control. In Canada the Jesuits deplored the fact that scarcely had they succeeded in converting the aborigines to Christianity than they were afflicted with disease and died in great numbers. In the *Jesuit Relations* of the time are such wistful entries as: "Hardly had they [the Indians] left Tadoussac—where they had listened with love to the Christian truths and presented their children for baptism—when death fell upon those little innocents, and disease upon a great part of their parents. There is no human eloquence which can persuade a people to embrace a Religion which seems to have for companions only pestilence, war and famine."

Samuel de Champlain, in 1615, estimated the population of the Hurons in eastern Canada to be more than thirty thousand. Although the center of population for this tribe was a comparatively small area between the Georgian Bay of Lake Huron and Lake Simcoe, their influence extended along the St. Lawrence valley as far as Quebec. Huron strength was instrumental in holding off the rival Iroquois, but the balance of power was soon to be altered by a new element. Contact with the whites brought disease, and of the situation in 1636 we read in *Jesuit Relations and Allied Documents,* edited by Edna Kenton: "The pestilence which for two years past had from time to time visited the Huron towns now returned with tenfold violence, and with it soon appeared a new and fearful scourge—the small pox. Terror was universal. The contagion increased as autumn advanced and when winter came, far from ceasing, its ravages were appalling."

In August of 1637 a meeting of Huron chiefs was held. The twofold crisis facing them demanded all their wisdom.

On one hand the destruction due to disease threatened their tribe with annihilation, on the other hand the scalping parties of the Iroquois harried the outskirts of their towns and killed Hurons in their forests and fields. They weathered this exigency, however, and by incorporating fragments of kindred tribes which in part made up their losses, they were believed by the French to have a population of upward of twenty thousand by 1639.

The respite was brief. The return of the epidemics was decisive, and by 1645 the destruction of the Hurons was complete. This time the best of their warriors were the victims and the Iroquois were quick to seize the advantage. In this fashion smallpox upset the entire balance of power between the Hurons and the Iroquois, destroying the former and at the same time signaling the failure of that Jesuit mission in Canada. The Hurons had frequently been difficult to convert; the Iroquois flatly refused to listen or to learn.

In between the North American settlements of France and Spain were those of England. Here a parallel situation existed. For several years prior to the arrival of the Pilgrims at Plymouth there had been a variety of explorations and fishing expeditions along the New England coast. In 1602 Bartholomew Gosnold had visited Martha's Vineyard and Cuttyhunk. Three years later Champlain explored the New England coast from Mount Desert to Cape Cod. There were other voyages including occasional raiding parties sent out to capture natives for slavery. There was ample opportunity for imported contagion to attack the New England Indians, either with contact with these various sorties or by an overland approach from Canada. Needless to say, the microorganisms did not overlook their advantage.

When Champlain dropped anchor at Cape Cod in 1605 he made note of the fact that there was a fairly dense indigenous population inhabiting the area. Fifteen years later, when the Pilgrims landed, the natives on the Cape and along the shoreline were relatively sparse. The reason for this disparity was a furiously violent epidemic occurring in 1617. The nature of this affliction has long been a debatable point. Many have assumed that it was smallpox, and probably the weight of the evidence would be in favor of this disease. Some believe that it may have been bubonic plague, but this is largely due to the fact that the epidemic was later referred to as "a plague." In the seventeenth century the term "plague" was even less specific than it is now. There are some adherents to the idea that yellow fever may have been the villain. This is a possibility but is very unlikely. At this distance the argument is academic, but the results for the English colonists were most significant.

The summer after the Pilgrims landed they sent two envoys on a diplomatic mission to treat with Massasoit, a famous chief encamped some forty miles away at what is now Warren, Rhode Island. The envoys discovered and described a scene of absolute havoc. Villages lay in ruins because there was no one to tend them. The ground was strewn with the skulls and the bones of thousands of Indians who had died and none was left to bury them. The Pilgrims in their own inimitable manner simply took it for granted that God smote the savages in order to make room for them.

Originally the Pilgrims had learned of this disaster from Samoset, an Indian from "down east" who had acquired a smattering of English from various explorers frequenting the Maine coast. Another informant was Squanto, a member of the Patuxit tribe previously dwelling in the area around Plymouth. Squanto, with about twenty other tribesmen, had been captured several years earlier by a slave raider and sold in Malaga. He managed to escape, eventually made his way to England, and succeeded in shipping home with Captain Thomas Dermer in 1619, only to make the horrifying discovery on his return that he was the sole member of his village still alive. All the others had perished in the epidemic two years before.

Following the establishment of the Plymouth and the

Massachusetts Bay colonies there were several epidemics, unquestionably of smallpox, among the natives. In 1631 a difference of opinion developed between the new Americans and the old. This was promptly settled to the complete satisfaction of Increase Mather who described the event some years later. According to the Reverend the natives became quarrelsome and began encroaching on the lands the settlers claimed to have purchased. "But," as Mather loftily remarks, "God ended the controversy by sending the small pox amongst the Indians at Saugust, who were before that time exceeding numerous. Whole towns of them were swept away, in some of them not so much as one Soul escaping the Destruction."

In 1634 we find John Winthrop writing to a friend in England, "But for the natives in these pts, God hath so pursued them, as for 300 miles space the greatest pte of them are swept awaye by the small poxe wch still continues among them: So as God hathe thereby cleered or title to this place, & those who remaine in these pts, being in all not 50, have putt themselves under or protection & freely confined themselves & their interest within certaine limitts."

In the same year the Connecticut Valley was the scene of a devastating epidemic. By this time the Dutch had established a trading post on the present site of Hartford, whereas members of the Plymouth Colony, much to the annoyance of the Hollanders, had planted one of their own a few miles upriver at Windsor. Governor Bradford tells the story:

> There was a company of people [Indians] lived in the country up above in the River of Connecticut a great way from their trading house there, and were enemies to those Indians which lived about them, and of whom they stood in some fear, being a stout people. About a thousand of them had enclosed themselves in a fort which they had strongly palisadoed about. Three or four Dutchmen went up in the beginning of winter to live with them, to get their trade and prevent them for bringing it to the English or to fall into amity with them: but at spring to bring all down to their place. But their enterprise failed. For it pleased God to visit

these Indians with a great sickness and such mortality that of a
thousand, above nine and a half hundred of them died, and many
of them did rot above ground for want of burial.

The Dutchmen themselves, nearly starved and frozen,
were glad to escape with their lives.

The virus also escaped alive, and soon the area around
the English post at Windsor was a terrifying spectacle.
Again from Bradford:

This spring also, those Indians that lived about their trading
house there, fell sick of the small pox and died most miserably;
for a sorer disease cannot befall them, they fear it more than the
plague. For usually they that have this disease have them in
abundance, and for want of bedding and linen and other helps
they fall into a lamentable condition as they lie on their hard
mats, the pox breaking and mattering and running one into
another, their skin cleaving by reason thereof to the mats they lie
on. When they turn them, a whole side will flay off at once as it
were, and they will be all of a gore blood, most fearful to behold.
And then being very sore, what with cold and other distempers,
they die like rotten sheep.

The conclusion is inescapable that the English, the
French, and the Spanish were materially aided in establishing a beachhead in the New World by the infections
they unwittingly introduced to a virgin area. Actually this
was probably the determining factor that spelled for them
the difference between success and failure. The natives, at
full strength, doubtless would have flung the invaders
back into the sea. As it was they melted away before a force
they could neither combat nor comprehend. Their incanta-
tions could not thwart it, nor their wampum influence it.
Nor, as we shall see, was its havoc to be confined to the
invasion coast. They were to be hounded in the mountains,
in the valleys, and on the plains until, except for scattered
remnants, they would vanish from the earth.

COUNTERATTACK

Although the newly imported ailments to which the
natives were suddenly exposed caused wholesale destruc-

tion among them, it would be entirely misleading to imply that disease held no terror for the invader as well. This factor was one of the major influences pinning him close to tidewater, and to the banks of the great inland waterways, for more than the next two hundred years. Although the death toll among the vigorous colonists during that period by no means approached the population growth from natural increase coupled with migration from abroad, it was still sufficient to inhibit any major expansion into the heartland. Sometimes the afflictions suffered were similar to those borne by the natives, sometimes the Europeans had troubles of their own.

• Within thirty years following the first voyage of Columbus, nearly all the West Indies as well as the connecting isthmus between the two American continents had been explored. To a large extent they had also been conquered and plundered by the Spaniards. In the area north of the Gulf of Mexico, however, very few discoveries had been made. It was no wonder that those fortunate adventurers who had amassed great riches in Mexico and Peru would dream of applying the same Midas touch to the vast and forbidding territory called Florida. But here, instead of gold and precious stones, they found belligerent savages and a trackless wilderness. Rather than high adventure and glory, there was frustration, disease, and death.

The first attempt at colonization by the Spanish in what is now continental United States was by Ponce de Leon in 1521. In the characteristic Spanish style, he brought clergymen for the colonists and friars to found Indian missions; and his supplies included horses, cattle, sheep, and swine. It was far better preparation than some founders had shown, but we have little reason to believe that there was anyone in the group with the slightest interest in growing from the soil anything that might sustain either the animals or the colonists, while the latter pursued their avid search for gold. Precisely where they struck the Florida coast we cannot be sure. Wherever it may have been, when they attempted to build dwellings the natives took a dim view, and Ponce de Leon, while leading his men against an uprising by the local residents, was wounded by an arrow. This was disheartening but not decisive. Shortly thereafter many of the settlers developed an illness undiagnosed up to now but severe enough to undermine morale, and the entire company fled to Cuba.

In 1526 another adventurer, Lucas Vasquez de Ayllon, sailed into Chesapeake Bay and up the first of the great rivers he encountered. He determined to make a settlement he named San Miguel at the same spot where, in the following century, the English would found Jamestown. On this point the Spanish erected shelters, using Negro slaves for the heaviest labor. These were the first bondmen to be introduced into the area that would become Virginia. Before the housing was completed winter came on, sickness broke out among the Europeans, and there were many deaths. Ayllon himself developed a pestilential fever and died on October 18, 1526. With the death of the leader there was chaos in the contingent. There were fracases with the Indians, the slaves became rebellious, and the colonists squabbled among themselves until it was finally resolved to abandon the enterprise. The initial attempts at colonization by the Spanish both in Florida and Virginia were dismal failures, and on both instances at least partially due to disease.

The epic travels of Hernando De Soto, who left Havana in May, 1539 with such confidence and glitter, ended with the explorer's death from a febrile illness, and the sullen Mississippi that he had discovered became his unmarked grave. One historian summed up the travails of De Soto's followers by saying, "I have not enumerated sickness and death among their sufferings, for these were the only comforts to their spirits, which sickened at the very thoughts of life." The feeble and intermittent grasp of Spain in these parts is in sharp contrast to the influence this nation exerted in the Southwest and in California.

Far to the north, meanwhile, the French too were probing into the unknown lands. In 1534 Jacques Cartier made a brief visit to Canada. It was enough to whet his appetite for a genuine voyage of exploration the following year. This was surely the expedition that would discover that long-sought passage to India.

On the tenth of May, 1535, Cartier set sail from the harbor of St. Malo with three tiny vessels. He crossed the stormy north Atlantic and spent some time exploring the great gulf that he named the Bay of St. Lawrence. Late that summer he sailed up the river soon to bear the same name. He paused and traded with the Indians camped beneath the frowning rock where Quebec now stands. Here, despite grave warnings from the natives of fearful perils awaiting upstream, he left two of his ships and with the smallest and a pair of open boats he pushed westward. He visited a large fortified Iroquois town at the foot of a great ridge, and then as autumn arrived he climbed and named the mountain of Montreal. Then he re-embarked and sailed back to the banks of the St. Charles River to make camp for the winter.

For several weeks all went well, then as the ice in the river thickened, and the snow on the banks grew deeper, disturbing rumors of disease came from the native villages. By December the French were aware that some fifty of the Indians had died. Cartier gave orders that the savages were not to approach either the fort or the ships, but despite these restrictions a strange illness began to appear among the newcomers. They lost their strength so that they could scarcely stand. Their legs became swollen. Black and blue marks appeared under the skin, and this without any injury to account for it. A most distressing condition appeared in the mouth. First the gums bled and then they literally rotted away so that the teeth fell out. Needless to say there was bad breath. There was an even worse situation from the defense point of view. By the middle of February Cartier noted ruefully that out of one hundred and ten of his people not more than ten were even in shape to give aid to the others. Eight were already dead and fifty more appeared to be dying.

The desperate plight of the explorers called for strong measures. At this juncture the first recorded autopsy in the Western Hemisphere was performed. Cartier apparently had no medical officer in his contingent, and it would have been amazing if he had. One sailor was discovered to possess some knowledge of surgery. Probably the poor man was himself ill at the time but regardless he was charged with the duty of "opening" a body. His report discussing the cause and results of the mortal illness of his subject was inconclusive, and many modern pathologists would empathize with his frustration.

The commander himself seemed to be more resistant to the affliction than the others. One day he went walking on the ice and encountered some Indians who appeared to be in fine shape. One in particular he knew had been very ill only a few days before, "his knees swelled as big as a child's head of two years old, his sinews shrunk, his teeth spoiled. . . ." Cartier was very casual in his inquiries because he had no intention of letting the natives know how forlorn his own situation was. The Indians readily told him that they were using a decoction made from the needles and bark of the spruce or the balsam fir. The disease of course was scurvy and the remedy was sovereign because here was an ample supply of ascorbic acid to effect an immediate cure. The sickly French promptly stripped and devoured the active ingredient from a whole tree, "and produced such a result, that had all the doctors of Louvain and Montpellier been there, with all the drugs of Alexandria, they could not have done so much in a year as did this tree in eight days."

A contemporary and rival of Cartier named Roberval had similar problems later in Canada. Although the two men together had planned the establishment of colonies in New France, apparently Cartier saw no reason to furnish his adversary with his own hard learned medical knowledge. As a result, Roberval at Cap Rouge on the St. Lawrence lost fifty of his men from scurvy during the winter of 1542.

The exigencies faced by the British in their earliest settlements were in many respects similar to those of the Spanish, and often for similar reasons—inadequate preparation, unrealistic motivation, and unadaptable personnel. Like the Spanish they were adventurers searching for riches to be had with minimum effort; like the Spanish their food supplies were insufficient for their most meager needs; and also, like the Spanish, they quarreled among themselves. They frequently went out of their way to enrage the savages, and they were unaccustomed to labor or hardship.

The original attempts at colonization were under the aegis of Sir Walter Raleigh on Roanoke Island off the coast of North Carolina. There is no evidence that the failure to found a permanent settlement either here or nearby was primarily due to disease, but other calamities intervened. Several years later the London Company obtained a charter from King James I bestowing on it a huge territory in North America and parlous days began.

To establish the initial colony in Virginia three vessels carrying one hundred and five settlers sailed in January 1607, and after following a somewhat devious course by the West Indies arrived in Chesapeake Bay late in April. There were two "chirurgeons" on board, which gave the medical profession a certain status among the ship's company, but more than half of the total complement were classed as "gentlemen" and the remainder as laborers and mechanics—not exactly the personnel required for a wilderness adventure.

One of the leaders of the expedition was John Smith, then twenty-eight years old. Smith arrived under something of a cloud because apparently on the voyage across the Atlantic his exuberance was interpreted by some as indicating mutiny. Another leader was Bartholomew Gosnold who had explored the New England coast five years earlier and who was far more knowledgeable about the country than any of the others. The ships anchored at a place named Point Comfort and a site for the colony was

selected about fifty miles inland from the mouth of the
James River on a point of land separated, in those days,
from the north bank by a marsh.

The new arrivals immediately set to work and by the
fifteenth of June a fort had been built, but disaster was
soon upon them. Sickness appeared and by September no
less than forty of the little band were dead. Most grievously
missed was Bartholomew Gosnold "vpon whose liefs stood
a great part of the good success and fortune of our gouer-
ment and Colony." By this time there were only six able
men in the community, but the leaders made certain that
the "savages" were not made aware of the desperate condition of the whites. The leaders even made a point of making sure that the colonists themselves were not acquainted
with the extent of their defenselessness.

The resourceful John Smith managed to barter some
corn from the Indians and so the struggling colony survived. During the winter a vessel appeared on the coast
with supplies and another contingent of settlers. When the
ship returned to England it carried a cargo of lumber, iron
ore, and sassafras. In those days when the science of
pharmacology was nearly as frenetic as it is now, the
volatile oil derived from the roots and bark of the sassafras
tree was considered to be a valuable remedy for syphilis,
dropsy, rheumatism, and most everything else.

Sassafras might just as well be exported. Assuredly it
would not cure the ailments then afflicting Jamestown.
The epidemic that originally struck the colony so viciously
that first summer was a violent dysentery, perhaps from
contaminated food, or water. Neither this nor the famine
which soon followed would yield to the roots and bark of
the trees of the forest. Once again there was hunger and
once again the diet of the Virginians was reduced to meal
and water. The population was cut in half by death before
the next relief ship arrived.

The following year was even worse. Grim experience
had taught the migrant English nothing. There was still no
consequential tillage of the soil. Fish and game were not

plentiful enough to support the company. One hungry husband took matters into his own hands, killed his wife and salted her down. According to contemporary accounts he feasted on his late mate roasted, boiled, and broiled. How his method of provisioning was discovered is not clear. Perhaps he invited some garrulous friends in for dinner. In any case he was executed and there was much comment about his poor taste both as a spouse and as a cook.

In 1610 Lord Delaware arrived in Virginia to take charge of the rapidly deteriorating situation. His abilities were of a high order and were desperately needed. Although he managed to rebuild and repair the village, his administration was very brief. Shortly after he landed he was seized with a violent fever which his physician, Dr. Laurence Bohun, cured by bloodletting. Soon after he regained his strength he relapsed. Following this, in turn he was assailed by "the Flux," then "the Cramps," and finally "the Gout." At this juncture the good lord became completely unstuck, developed scurvy, and decided he was about to leave the world. All he departed then, however, was the New World. He sailed for the West Indies, but due more to contrary winds than to faulty navigation he made a landfall in the Azores where a diet of "Orenges and Lemonds" produced a therapeutic triumph even more dramatic than that of Dr. Bohun's.

The principal health problems facing the Spaniards, the French, and the English in their earliest attempts at exploration and settlement in North America were not due to unfamiliar and potent microorganisms lying in wait for the unsuspecting Europeans. Rather they were the result of carelessness, unpreparedness, and ignorance on the part of the foreigner. Death among the first arrivals was primarily due to starvation, to self-contaminated food and water, and to scurvy. Starvation was as frequently due to lack of foresight and disinclination to manual labor as it was to misfortune. Contamination of food and water was in part due to laziness, in part to lack of any instinctive desire for simple cleanliness, and to utter ignorance of the basic rules of public health to be found in the Old Testament.

The incredible part of the story relates to scurvy. It may be unfair to be critical of Champlain or of the early settlers of Virginia because they were unfamiliar with methods for prevention and cure of this disease. Such methods had been discovered and described often enough in the previous century by the French, the English, and the Dutch to have become by then a part of folklore. Somehow it just did not happen. Time after time the immediate and unfailing response to evergreen needles, watercress, "scurvy grass," fresh fruits and vegetables, lemon juice, lime juice and various other substances was described. Yet it was nearly two hundred years before scurvy was eliminated even from the British navy.

LET MY PEOPLE GO

The importation of infectious disease to the western world was by no means wholly the work of the explorers and the colonists. Of great importance, too, were the infections introduced and reintroduced over a matter of centuries by the slave trade. Because of this commerce, orations without end, volumes without number, protests and prayers without stint poured forth over the years. Despite all this verbiage, the basic facts of the medical geography of the Americas and of Africa, on which the merchandizing of human lives was based, have largely been ignored.

The voyages of Columbus created a huge labor market. There was a whole new hemisphere to develop. In the mines, in the forests, and in the fields there was hard work to be done. It was a foregone conclusion that the Europeans were not going to do it. The natives, for the most part, were not going to do it either. Those who stood their ground and fought were killed by the invader. Those who stayed and submitted, lacking the necessary immunity, died promptly of his diseases. There was but one chance to survive, namely to flee, but even that opportunity was closed to the island dwellers.

As the sugar plantations developed with surprising speed in the Caribbean islands, there came a strident demand for Negroes direct from Africa. As these islands were taken over by the enterprising English, French, Dutch and Danes, there was increasing insistence on the need for slave labor, each nation recognizing the importance of retaining a foothold in Africa.

As the English colonies in North America progressed, they established a pattern of their own. Although it is usually thought that there was scant demand for slaves in the northern colonies where they were primarily employed only as domestic servants, the trade there could not have been inconsequential. A census taken in 1754 disclosed that there were 2,707 slaves in Massachusetts alone. It was, however, in the South where the great bulk of the slave population would reside. The warmer regions provided an abundance of tillable acreage, and the soil was suitable to the cultivation of tobacco, rice, and indigo, crops that could be grown profitably on a large scale and required much space and many laborers. Although cotton falls in the same category, its extensive cultivation in the South would have to await the ingenuity of a Connecticut Yankee.

Labor in colonial America was scarce and expensive for several reasons. A person with the initiative and the urge to migrate to a new and unsettled country was ordinarily the type of individual who would lead more readily than follow. The original settlers were not a laboring class except in the sense that some were farmers or artisans and therefore dependent on their own efforts to make a livelihood. They were not men who would cheerfully toil and sweat to enrich someone else. Furthermore it was apparent from the very beginning that the Indians could neither be hired nor forced to work in the fields because of their psychological and emotional make-up. Although there were many instances of captured Indians being sold as slaves, this traffic never became a large-scale operation. Indentured servants, Scotch and Irish who were captured in battle, or English lads who were conned into taking a free trip to America were sold from the time of the earliest settlements, but even this was on too small a scale to fill the needs of an expanding agriculture.

Early in colonial days Great Britain forbade the cultivation of tobacco in the British Isles, so that Maryland and Virginia had a virtual monopoly on its production. As a result, in the last four decades of the seventeenth century the tobacco colonies required an increasing number of slaves, and the only adequate supply came from Africa. Furthermore it was the Negro's relative immunity to malaria that made possible the development of rice plantations in South Carolina. The Negroes required "seasoning" because the climate and the food were unfamiliar, but those who had survived the hazards of their original habitat and the horrors of the Middle Passage might be counted on for many years of service.

The medical geography of the Americas, therefore, was a relatively simple environment made up of a large, fertile and healthful land to which the invader brought multitudes of malignant microorganisms before which the aborigines either fled or perished. The medical geography of Africa, on the other hand, was neither simple nor salubrious. On the contrary it was contained, contaminated, contagious, and complex.

The factors that made Africa "the dark continent" and "the white man's grave" were to have a profound influence on the history of the United States. These were the very factors that permitted, and enhanced, the forced emigration of several million natives with their diseases and immunities to the Western Hemisphere. The continent of Africa had been known by civilized people from earliest times, yet as late as the early decades of the nineteenth century only isolated sections of the west coast were known by Europeans. By this time the North American continent had been crossed and recrossed, the great rivers, the great plains, the great mountains and the great lakes had been explored, mapped and to some extent settled. The magnificent cataract at Niagara had been described two hundred years before Livingstone stood at Victoria Falls, and Lake Erie had been fought over by modern navies before Albert Nyanza even appeared on modern charts.

Then why was North America so thoroughly explored and exploited while Africa, no farther away from Europe than the Straits of Gibraltar, was to remain the dark continent until the past hundred years?

North Africa, the narrow zone lying between the Mediterranean Sea and the Sahara, is geologically a part of the Mediterranean region. The Sahara, lying under a searing sun, a vast terrain of gravel, rocks and sand, provides a formidable barrier between that landlocked sea and Central Africa. The natural approach to the continent, therefore, would appear to be along the thousands of miles of coastline, and this very idea occurred to Henry the Navigator of Portugal early in the fifteenth century, some years before Columbus was born.

The grim facts of geography and the even grimmer facts of biology militated against Henry's captains and those who were to follow in their stead. The coast of Africa, except along the Mediterranean, has almost no good harbors. Much of the shore is sandy beach with only shallow water to seaward, and the whole frequently protected by treacherous reefs. Seagoing vessels must anchor offshore and lighter in for their cargoes. The only approach below the Sahara leading inland was by the rivers. There were several of these large enough to accommodate for miles into the interior, vessels of considerable draft. But here appeared the most formidable barrier of all, more dismal than the dreary desert, more dangerous than the shallow shoreline—the impenetrable barricade of disease. Africa was the dark continent from time immemorial not because of the ferocity of the black man, not because of the wild beasts of the jungle, but rather because of such occasional afflictions as yaws, filariasis, and schistosomiasis, and especially because of such scourges as smallpox, yellow fever, dysentery, trypanosomiasis, and malaria.

It is absolutely impossible to be certain about the etiologic forces responsible for the ailments that occurred early in the trading days to Africa, but many accounts raise the suspicion of yellow fever. The voyages of Aluise Ca da Mosto, a Venetian nobleman in the service of Prince Henry, began in 1455. On his second voyage in 1456, "Having ascended the river Gambia for about sixty miles to the country of Battimansa, Ca da Mosto halted, sent a deputation to the chief, and received on board a large number of natives." The adventurer then makes the significant comment "at the end of the eleventh day we decided to leave and go to the mouth of the river, because many of us had begun to suffer with hot fever which is acute and continuous." The suspicion is strong that this might have been yellow fever. The same might be said of another commercial voyage, this one made by the British farther south to Benin in 1553 in which "scarcely forty" out of 140 men returned to Plymouth. Nearly all the deaths occurred within little more than a month aboard ship lying at the mouth of the Benin River, the men dying "sometimes three and sometimes four or five in a day." In a similar voyage to Benin in 1588, the loss was proportionately as great.

On the other side of the continent, the Nile Valley would appear to have offered a natural thoroughfare across the Sahara in early times, but at six different places the great river rushes through rocky gorges, and much more to be dreaded, beyond these navigational barriers was the far more unsurmountable obstacle of febrile disease. For years the Sudan was famed for its unhealthiness, and Egyptians long considered an order to serve in its desert wastes, and still more in its distant equatorial provinces, as tantamount to a death sentence.

Along the Upper Nile there existed a particularly viru-

lent form of smallpox. One who encountered this problem
was a Scotchman named James Bruce, who in the latter
half of the eighteenth century had set himself the objective
of discovering the source of the Nile. When Bruce
appeared at Gondar, the capital of Abyssinia, he found
several of the leading citizens were ill with smallpox.
Although Bruce had less therapeutic background than the
most recent graduate among the native medicine men, two
deaths in the carriage trade in Gondar coupled with the
Britisher's confident bedside manner assured him of a
chance to prescribe for the remaining patients. Since these
were on the way to recovery anyway, Bruce reaped the
reward that self-limited diseases have bestowed on many
practitioners, trained and untrained.

Bruce gained such favor at court that he was allowed
to continue with guides to the source of the Blue Nile,
reaching there in 1770, long after its original discovery by
a Portuguese priest. On his return to Gondar, Bruce was
prostrated by some type of fever from which he recovered
and went home to Scotland where he died at the age of
sixty-four by falling down his own stairs and landing on his
head. This demise hardly warrants recording here except
to note that Bruce failed to establish a precedent among
African explorers for dying at home. There were very few
others who did.

It is noteworthy that among the early British explorers
there was a rather high proportion of physicians who abandoned their patients to trudge through the fever-ridden
swamps of Africa. Perhaps even before the present-day
panel system, the practice of medicine in Britain left something to be desired. The first of these peripatetic practitioners was Mungo Park, who made an initial and exciting trip
to Africa in 1795. Following his roundabout return home
he settled at Peebles and practiced surgery for a couple of
years, but the call of the jungle was more enticing than the
abscesses and amputations of a tiny Scottish village. He
determined to retrace his steps up the Gambia a considerable distance, strike off across country to the Niger, and

then go downstream to the ocean. Park's last dispatches were from Sansandig, on the Niger, and he says, "I am sorry to say that of forty-four Europeans who left the Gambia in perfect health, five only are at present alive; viz, three soldiers (one deranged in his mind), Lieutenant Maclyn and myself. . . . We had no contest with the natives, nor was any of us killed by wild animals or any other accident." So the good doctor left Sansandig on the nineteenth of November, 1805, and later it was learned that his boat had struck a rock on the way downstream. While the party were reconnoitering the rapids and trying to avoid unfriendly natives on the bank, they plunged overside and were drowned in the river they were attempting to explore.

The morbidity and mortality among the early nineteenth century explorers were enormous. Sir Samuel Baker took his bride along his jaunt to Lake Albert, and at one point she was attacked with "gastric fever" (typhoid?). He was prostrated with ague, and at the same time they were in the vicinity of a group of slave-hunting Turks among whom smallpox was rife. Another early explorer was a German, Frederick Conrad Horneman, who traveled from Cairo to Murzuk in what is now Libya, where he remained for some time because of illness. On his return to Tripoli he died of a fever. A venturesome Swiss, John Louis Burckhardt, went up the Nile nearly to Dongola, and later, disguised as an Arab, traveled east, all the way to Mecca, but returned only to die in Cairo at the age of twenty-two.

From England, Hugh Clapperton signed on for an expedition with Dr. Oudney and Colonel Denham. They reached Lake Chad in February, 1823, but Dr. Oudney died before they had gone much farther. Clapperton returned to England and soon was off on another expedition to strike inland from the mouth of the Benin River. This time he accompanied Captain Pearce of the Royal Navy, Mr. Dickson, a surgeon, and another Navy surgeon and naturalist, Dr. Morrison. They started inland in December, 1825, and for some reason Dickson left the others and was afterwards killed. Within a few days Clapperton had chills and fever but kept on with the party. Pearce died on December twenty-seventh and Dr. Morrison succumbed on the following day. Clapperton went on and made important discoveries, but died of dysentery in northwestern Nigeria in April, 1827. Colonel Denham, mentioned previously, died of a fever in Sierra Leone in June, 1828.

James Kingston Tuckey was an Irishman who survived nine years of captivity by the French during the Napoleonic Wars. Following his release he was selected by the British government to command an expedition to the Congo River. In 1816 Captain Tuckey succeeded in ascending the river some 280 miles, but not much information was obtained and Tuckey died before the year was out.

In May, 1841, an expedition set sail from England that was intended to settle, once and for all, the long disputed geography of the Niger River. Captain Henry Dundas Trotter, with three steamers fully equipped for such an enterprise, entered the mouth of the fateful stream on August 13th. In less than three weeks the passengers on two of the vessels were so utterly incapacitated by raging fever that they could do nothing but turn back downstream. Trotter, in the *Albert*, struggled on for some distance, but by October third the commander was himself prostrated by fever, and there was nothing to do but turn back. The Niger was not yet willing to reveal her secrets.

On Stanley's expedition to find Dr. Livingstone, the intrepid reporter was himself delayed by no less than twenty-three attacks of fever in the thirteen months that the journey lasted. Many of these febrile episodes were literally so severe and prolonged that he was actually unconscious for many weeks. On this journey, so famous and yet so unimportant considering those Stanley would later make, he would find that dysentery, elephantiasis, smallpox, and a host of other ailments would serve to render many of his men physically helpless, and even more important, emotionally demoralized.

In 1734 a British naval surgeon, John Atkins, described a type of sleeping sickness he had observed on the Guinea coast:

> The Sleepy Distemper (common among the Negroes) gives no other previous Notice, than a want of Appetite 2 or 3 days before; their sleeps are sound, and Sense and Feeling very little; for pulling drubbing or whipping will scarce stir up Sense and Power enough to move; and the Moment you cease beating the smart is forgot, and down they fall again into a state of Insensibility, drivling constantly from the Mouth as if in deep salivation; breathe slowly, but not unequally nor snort. Young people are more subject to it than the Old; and the Judgment generally pronounced is Death, the Progsnotick seldom failing. If now and then one of them recovers, he certainly loses the little Reason he had, and turns Ideot. . . .

African sleeping sickness was known for centuries before its etiology was understood. Slave traders in early years came to recognize the symptoms of lethargy among Negroes and the risks and high mortality of the infection. They also perceived, long before Winterbottom described them in 1803, that the swollen posterior cervical glands of the Negro were an ominous sign, and refused to purchase such individuals. In the literature of the slave trade are such comments as, "Whydah Slaves are more subject to Small-Pox and sore Eyes; other parts to a sleepy Distemper. . . ." or else, "Mr. Knox in the *Sherbro* purchased but 13 Slaves in 3 Months time, and two of them died of the Lethargy Soon after."

The cause of African sleeping sickness is neither a virus nor a species of bacteria, but, like malaria, is due to a variety of protozoa, in this case a trypanosome. It is transmitted to man and to domestic animals by the bite of a brownish insect, the tsetse fly that breeds in the lush foliage close by the banks of African rivers. Trypanosomiasis has long been an absolute scourge affecting not only the natives but also the explorer, as well as killing his beasts of burden and thwarting his journeys of discovery. Furthermore, the economic losses from the destruction of

livestock frustrated those who attempted agricultural development in the hinterland. This disease has had a profound effect on the medical geography of Africa and has
been one of the blackest clouds overhanging the continent.

So there were smallpox, yellow fever, and trypanosomiasis; there were typhoid and dysentery; there were yaws
and schistosomiasis and filariasis; but of all the morbid
threats to those who would storm the bastions of Festung
Africa, the greatest was malaria. It was prevalent in the
basins of the Senegal and the Gambia, along the whole
Guinea coast from Sierra Leone and in the basins of the
Niger and the Gabon and down the coast to Cape Lopez,
and again in Benguela. On the east coast from the Lim-
popo to the Zambesi, in Mozambique and Zanzibar, inland
beyond Lake Ngami and at Massawa, there was malaria.
Malaria extended from the Abyssinian highlands across
the Sudan, north along the Nile, westward to Lake Chad,
and again in Tripoli, Tunis, and Algiers.

In 1849 a British physician, Dr. William F. Daniell
wrote, "Were it not for the fatal insalubrity of climate, so
deleterious to the European constitution where life is not
forfeited at once, it is impossible to say what extent our
commercial intercourse would have acquired with the inland regions of the vast continent of Africa which lie at this
moment unexplored and unknown." It is this very situation which made it possible for the slave trade to continue
for the centuries that it did. If there had been no significant dangers in Africa other than those of deserts, mountains, wild beasts, and inhospitable natives, the region
would have swarmed with explorers by the beginning of
the seventeenth century. These would have been followed
by settlers, wars, and civilization—but not by the slave
trade. Under these circumstances it would have been impossible for the local black potentates along the coast to
send raiding parties inland to capture and sell to offshore
slavers huge numbers of Negroes of both sexes and all
ages. The manpower would not have been available to
make the raids, nor would the victims have been un-

equipped with firearms. The cost of procuring slaves would have been prohibitive.

Although the medical geography of the Americas and Africa made the slave trade possible, there is no point in speculating on what would have been the case if the situations had been different. The slave trade did occur, and it had a most significant impact on the medical history of this country.

The largest slave market, and therefore the greatest problem area, was South Carolina. In Charlestown (as it was then spelled), attempts were made as early as 1698 to establish a feeble quarantine mechanism. The previous year there had been much smallpox with a high fatality rate not only in the town but among the Pemlico Indians. In 1699 yellow fever made its first appearance, killing 160 persons and continuing as an intermittent threat to the health of the neighborhood for the next two hundred years.

In 1711 one writer described the situation in no uncertain terms, "Never was there a more sickly or fatall season than this for small Pox, Pestilential Ffeavers, Pleurisies, and fflux's have destroyed great numbers here of all Sorts, both Whites Blacks and Indians. . . ." The shambles brought action by the General Assembly of South Carolina, and in 1712, "Whereas great Numbers of the Inhabitants of this Province have been Destroyed by Malignant, Contagious Diseases Brought here from Africa, and other Parts of America. . . ." Gilbert Guttery was appointed as "a Commissioner for Enquiring into the State of health of all Such persons as Shall be aboard Any Ship or Vessell Arriveing in this Province." His duties were to visit all vessels before anyone else was allowed on board, to order masters to send their sick to the pest house, and hold vessels in quarantine for twenty days if anyone on board had died of a contagious disease. This was a perfectly sound and sensible arrangement, and probably was far more effective than was then realized, but errors could be made as is indicated by a news item in the *South Carolina Gazette* for May 4, 1738, "Several of the Negroes imported in the Ship London Frigate, which arrived here the 13th of April last, have been since discovered to have the small Pox, there are few of them in Town but more in the Country and several were sent on board again, the ship having been ordered to fall down to the Fort to perform Quarentine."

But it was too late, and the result was a terrific epidemic among those dwelling in the town and the surrounding countryside which promptly spread among the neighboring Indians, destroying almost half of the Cherokee nation within the next year.

The experience of this tragic visitation could not help but result in public health action, and as a consequence more stringent measures were applied and a new pest house was built on Sullivan's Island.

African trypanosomiasis was not exported to the New World because the tsetse fly refused to leave home. There seems to be little doubt that hookworm disease came along with the slaves and established itself here to such an extent that the causative agent was named *Necator americanus*. Nevertheless, despite our chauvinistic desires, the worm appears to have originated in Africa. Filariasis became established in a small endemic focus near Charleston, the only one in the United States, and did not die out until the twentieth century. Similarly, leprosy appeared along the Gulf coast, presumably brought in with slaves. But of far greater significance was the fact that time after time the coastal towns of what is now the United States were reinfected with yellow fever, smallpox, dysentery, and malaria reintroduced by the slave trade. If it is true that the gods visit the sins of the fathers upon the children, ours has been a lethal legacy.

THE MOPPING UP

It is difficult for either the modern physician or layman, accustomed as he is to the ubiquitous spectre of disease, to be credulous of a health situation so salubrious as that described by William Wood, one of our original realtors. Wood was an Englishman who came to New England in 1623 and returned home ten years later to write a lengthy commercial to induce his countrymen to settle in the new land. He has this to say of the health of the natives, "The Indians be of lusty and healthfull bodies, not experimentally knowing the Catalogue of those health-wasting diseases which are incident to other countries, as Feavers, Pleurisies, Callentures, Agues, Obstructions, Consumptions, Subfumigations, Convulsions, Apoplexies, Dropsies, Gouts, Stones, Toothaches, Pox, Measels or the like but spinne out the thread of their dayes to a faire length, numbering three-score, four-score, some a hundred years, before the world's Universall summoner cite them to the craving Grave."

Later he claimed never to have seen "one that was borne either in redundance or defect a monster, or any that sickness had deformed, or casualtie made decrepit, saving one that had a bleared eye and an other that had a wenne on his cheek." This should hardly be taken as evidence that congenital defects or crippling disease did not occur. Inasmuch as the antics of the medicine men would scarcely prolong the lives of such victims, and tribal existence was not compatible with nursing home techniques, it is reasonable to assume that these unfortunates merely died before Mr. Wood made his rounds.

On the whole, however, Wood was probably right, and although the bulk of the evidence is negative and deals for the most part with the ailments the aborigines did not have, still the weight of informed opinion seems to be on his side.

Colonel P. M. Ashburn, who spent many years studying the matter, is forthright in his conclusions: "Prior to the coming of the white man and the Negro, America was a land almost free from infectious diseases. Death on the wholesale scale came only from war, drought, flood and famine, and on the small scale mainly from accidents and injuries, the mishaps and complications of childbearing,

the sacrifice of captives and old age." A similar conclusion is reached by the distinguished anthropologist Dr.
Ales Hrdlicka, who makes no bones about it.

> Before America was discovered by Columbus it was apparently
> one of the—if not the—most healthful continents. We may judge
> of this by the relative richness of the population in all the regions
> when discovered. There were no areas depopulated by disease,
> and the early white settlers witnessed, it would seem, no
> epidemics that were of purely American origin. The skeletal re-
> mains of unquestionably precolumbian date are, barring a few
> exceptions, remarkably free from disease. Whole important
> scourges were wholly unknown. There was no rachitis; there was
> no tuberculosis. There was no pathologic microcephaly, no hydro-
> cephaly. There was no plague, cholera, typhus, smallpox or
> measles. Cancer was rare, and even fractures were infrequent.
> There was no lepra. Notwithstanding some claims to the con-
> trary, there is as yet not a single instance of thoroughly authenti-
> cated precolumbian syphilis. . . .

So the newcomers, white and black, were responsible
for the introduction to an entire continent of malaria and
yellow fever, of smallpox, typhus, typhoid and scarlet fever,
of dengue, diphtheria, measles and whooping cough, of
gonorrhea and syphilis and of cholera and tuberculosis.

The advance agents of civilization were well armed,
better than they knew, and the aborigines were defenseless, much more than they realized. Under the circumstances, dealing as we are with a continent, a scattered
population and a time lapse of four and one-half centuries,
it is difficult to weave an organized story of the demise of a
race. Some of the events of the early years have already
been detailed, and now we must describe cursorily a number of unrelated events—unrelated in time and location—which nevertheless eventually came to be related
inexorably to the ultimate destruction of a people. It is all
very well to say that there are still many thousands of
Indians within our borders, huddling on reservations and
dependent on Congressional largesse. But the fact remains
that as a *people* they are dead, and they died of imported
disease.

The greatest killer of all was smallpox. The Indian apparently had almost no immunity to the disease. He was habitually sociable, living crowded together in wigwams, hogans, or dugouts; he had no concept of sanitation or quarantine, and his migratory tendencies in search of food led him into constant contact with other villages. All these elements inevitably produced a major conflagration from a single spark. Many of the outbreaks in Canada, New England and New York occurring in early colonial days are mentioned elsewhere in this volume. In 1731, an epidemic among the Senecas in eastern Canada produced such terror that they fled to Massachusetts and New Hampshire and effectually spread the malady throughout the Six Nations. Peter Kalm, traveling through Pennsylvania, New Jersey, and New York in 1749–50, was impressed by the incredible number of deaths among the Indians due to smallpox.

The introduction of the virus among the Indians may not always have been accidental. During the war with Pontiac in 1763 that famed soldier of the king, Sir Jeffrey Amherst, wrote a suggestion to Colonel Bouquet, "Could it not be contrived to send the Small Pox among those disaffected tribes of Indians? We must on this occasion use every strategem in our power to reduce them." Bouquet was prompt to reply, "I will try to inoculate the —— with some blankets that may fall in their hands, and take care not to get the disease myself." Inasmuch as smallpox had broken out at Fort Pitt at the time, this was an entirely practical plan. Whether it was actually carried out or not we do not know, but the following spring the disease was prevalent among Mingoes, Delawares, and Shawanoes in the vicinity.

In 1774 there were only 1,363 Indians in Connecticut and 1,432 in Rhode Island. Regarding the situation farther south, the Reverend Elam Potter of New Haven had gathered statistics on this matter and had written to Dr. Ezra Stiles September 12, 1768, stating of the Cherokees, "The Rev. Mr. Richardson of South Carolina informs me, that when he was amongst them as a missionary, ten years ago, they had about 1500 fighting men; but since then they have been greatly diminished by the wars with other nations, with the English, and by the small pox, which is a most fatal disease among them." Of the Cataupas (Cataw-bas), "These are a nation who lie upon the river Cataupa near the line that divides North and South-Carolina . . . They live upon a tract . . . which was to consist of 30 miles square. In the year 1760 they were so reduced by the small pox that they have accepted of but 15 miles square. They may consist of 20 or 30 families, and their number is about 100 souls."

It would appear that between 1740 and 1770 the dec-imation among the Indians dwelling along the eastern seaboard was so severe that these tribes were far too impo-tent to play a significant part in the Revolution on either side in that entire area.

Similar situations were occurring elsewhere on the continent. An outbreak that developed in western Canada about 1780 was in this fashion described by Alexander MacKenzie:

> In short, it appeared, that the natives had formed a resolution to extirpate the traders . . . and nothing but the greatest calamity that could have befallen the natives, saved the traders from de-struction: this was the small-pox, which spread its destructive and desolating power, as the fire consumes the dry grass of the field. The fatal infection spread around with a baneful rapidity which no flight could escape, and with a fatal effect that nothing could resist. It destroyed with its pestilential breath whole families and tribes; . . .

The turn of the nineteenth century was to bring no surcease, as the following extract from the Lewis and Clark journals will testify:

> 14th August Tuesday 1804
> The men Sent to the Mahar Town last evining has not returned we Conclude to send a Spye to Know the Cause of their delay, at about 12 oClock the Party returned and informed. us that they Could not find the Indians, nor any fresh Sign, those people have

not returned from their Buffalow hunt. Those people haveing no houses no Corn or anything more than the graves of their ansesters to attach them to the old Village, Continue in purseute of the Buffalow longer than others who has greater attachments to their native village. The ravages of the Small Pox (which Swept off 400 men & Womin & childred in perpopotion) has reduced this nation not exceeding 300 men and left them to the insults of their weaker neighbours, which before was glad to be on friendly turms with them. I am told when this fatal malady was among them they Carried their franzey to verry extroadinary length, not only of burning their Village, but they put their wives & children to Death with a view of their all going together to some better Countrey. they burry their Dead on the top of high hills and rais Mounds on top of them. The cause or way those people took the Small Pox is uncertain, the most Probable, from Some other nation by means of a warparty.

One official report to the secretary of war states that smallpox in 1802 destroyed half the population from the Missouri River to New Mexico in the region of the Pawnees and thence west to the Rockies.

After the epidemic of 1801–02 had run its course, no serious outbreak seems to have occurred in the Indian population for some thirteen years. However, in 1815–16 a most virulent eruption appeared among all the tribes along the Red and the Rio Grande rivers in the Southwest. Presumably it originated in and was imported from the Spanish settlements, as were so many of the scourges among the Southwestern tribes of the United States. According to their own account, the Comanches alone lost four thousand of their people.

About 1831 another episode in our tumultuous relationship with the Indians was taking place. It is one in which we can take no pride, and for that reason gets scant attention in the history books. In the early years of the nineteenth century, when settlers began migrating in large numbers into the southeastern and south central states, they found native tribes quite unlike those encountered elsewhere in this country. These were not wandering, hunting nomads, continually on the warpath. They had lived in the same valleys and along the same streams for years, perhaps for centuries. They built permanent homes, and grew crops including cotton that they carded and wove into cloth for clothing.

But the fact remains they were in the way of civilization, and progress, of the nineteenth century. The election of Andrew Jackson sealed their doom, and what had been a haphazard undertaking now became a firm policy. Within little more than a decade, sixty thousand Indians—men, women and children—were to be torn from their homes and forced to travel, to be dumped on the far side of the Mississippi River, there to shift for themselves.

Untold numbers never arrived at their earthly Promised Land. They died of smallpox and measles, of Asiatic cholera and malaria. They died of starvation and alcoholism. Cherokees died in Georgia, Creeks died in Alabama, Choctaws and Chickasaws died in Arkansas. Scarce wonder that they themselves called it the Trail of Tears.

History does not represent everything that has happened to the human race, but only what has been recorded about these events. Our knowledge of the history of the American Indians depends almost entirely on what white people wrote. The unwritten history of the Indians must contain countless forgotten stories of heroism, misery, sacrifice, disease, and death even in recent times. Thousands of the American aborigines, minding their own business in the first half of the nineteenth century, found themselves and their children suddenly struck with a fever, a fearful rash of pustular areas on the skin, often a delirium, and no surcease but to crawl into a hole or leap into a stream and die.

The most thoroughly documented, and therefore what we are inclined to interpret as the worst, epidemic of smallpox to assail the Indians during the nineteenth century in North America was first recorded in this fashion, "Friday 14—One of the warmest days that we have had this summer—Weather smokey—A young Mandan died to day of the Small Pox—several others has caught it—the Indians all being out Makeing dried Meat has saved several of them."

This was the entry of Friday, July 14, 1837, in the journal of Francis A. Chardon, a fur trader at Fort Clark, a trading post of the American Fur Company built six years earlier on the west bank of the Upper Missouri about fifty-five miles above Bismarck, North Dakota. Nearly a month before, the little steamer *St. Peter's,* on her annual spring trip from St. Louis to collect buffalo robes and beaver skins, had bartered with lethal coin. There was smallpox on board the vessel, and soon there was smallpox ashore.

Early explorers to the area had found the Mandans to be a populous and potent people, but some fifty-five years before its appearance at Fort Clark, smallpox had dealt the tribe a shattering blow. At that time war parties from the south had brought the disease with them to areas where it had never been before. From some nine villages the Mandans had been reduced to two, and because of their military impotence had withdrawn from the country near what is now Bismarck to the northwest. The Mandans were never a vigorous people again. In one entry Chardon sneered, "Brave Warriors as Dayvy Crocrite says, in time of Peace." Certainly they were not a serious threat to other Indians, but their numbers had increased and they were carrying on a relatively active trade with the fur company. The visit of the *St. Peter's* literally annihilated them. A tribe consisting of some 1,600 persons was reduced to 31 souls.

But that was not all. Other tribes for hundreds of miles were desperately involved. There were the Minnetarees and the Arickarees who were reduced by half, the Assiniboins who were even more severely attacked, and then the Pawnees who had vivid memories of their epidemic of six years earlier, were re-infected from some Oglala women and children they had captured, and again the Pawnees lost about a quarter of their tribe. The Crees and particularly the Blackfeet suffered enormously in this epidemic.

Obviously, at this time no census had ever been taken of the Plains Indians. Also, the actual mortality that occurred in those ghastly final months of 1837 is mere guesswork. A very conservative estimate is that something more than 17,000 Indians in the Northwest died in a matter of months. And so it was recorded, "In whatever direction you turn, nothing but sad wrecks of mortality meet the eye: lodges standing on every hill, but not a streak of smoke rising from them. Not a sound can be heard to break the awful stillness, save the ominous croak of ravens, and the mournful howl of wolves, fattening on the human carcasses that lie strewed around." All this could not help but exert great influence not merely on tribal relationships in the Northwest, but equally on the balance of power between Indian and white. With the destruction of Indian military potential by disease, the opportunities for settlement were greatly increased and vastly simplified.

There were two other serious problems which, partly because of lack of any useful data and partly because of built-in embarrassments, we tend to sweep under the rug. The first of these, and one there is little point in spending much time on, is venereal disease.

The reason for slighting the subject is not because of prudishness, but because of lack of data. The present writer is not of the school that believes that "Columbus discovered syphilis in 1492," but rather contends along with Hrdlicka that "Syphilis in such form as it now exists among white races and in the Indian or Eskimo infected by the white man or the Negro did not, in all probability, exist in precolumbian America." Furthermore, it is difficult enough to develop useful public health information regarding this topic in a civilized, presumably controlled, modern population, so that any data regarding aborigines is utterly invalid.

The Lewis and Clark Journals do offer one sidelight on the issue. "January 27th 1806. Goodrich has recovered from the Louis Veneri which he contracted from an amorous contact with a Chinnook damsel, I cured him as I did

Gibson last winter by the use of mercury." Poor Goodrich!
He probably contracted his disease from one of the very
few possible sources then extant in the Northwest, but
there she was!

There is little more factual information of genuine
value available regarding alcohol, but here perhaps the
situation is even more tragic. In the first place the whiskey
provided was almost always done so illegally, and invariably as the result of avarice and malice on the part of the
whites. This is not the occasion to delve deeply either into
the physiopathology, or even less, into the sociology of
alcohol. Doubtless the stuff sold or given to the Indians
was raw and potent by any standards. Furthermore, drinking was almost universal and drunkenness was commonplace along the frontier. The unfortunate facts were that
alcohol was made available to the Indians with more ominous aims in view than merely to extend sociability or even
as a convenient substitute for coin. Treaties were signed,
bargains were driven, and suicides initiated with its invalu-
able assistance. The Indian had no more resistance to the
effects of alcohol than he had to pathogenic bacteria, and
as is the case with many primitive peoples, he frequently
went berserk under its influence. All inhibitions were dis-
solved. The Indian frequently became crazed, and oftentimes literally drank himself to death. As has been inti-
mated, no statistics are available, but although the data is
meager, the true mortality was doubtless considerable and
the morbidity was greater yet.

So east and west, north and south, the grim spectre of
disease haunted the natives. Smallpox, dysentery, venereal
disease, and many other afflictions time and again devastated the savage population. But then an unexpected invader, although perhaps a familiar acquaintance in these
pages, was suddenly to appear, wreak havoc upon the
tribes and exert a telling influence on the future of the
Northwest. This was malaria.

Well, was it malaria? Frequently a dubious cry is
raised, and in some circles even now an argument will be

forthcoming. The mortality among the savages was far too high. It is unbelievable that so many should die so abruptly of this affliction. Much more likely that pandemic influenza or scarlet fever or typhus or typhoid was responsible. Doubtless there were other infections current at the time, and some fatalities were caused by organisms other than the plasmodium, but the case for malaria in the present-day attempt to unravel yesterday's mysteries is still good.

In the first place, the contemporary accounts continually refer to "fever and ague," and "ague" implies a chill that would rattle the tepee. The distribution was overwhelmingly in the valleys and along the coast. It occurred during the warm weather. Malaria-bearing mosquitoes are known to exist in the locality. Finally, although the mortality among the natives was phenomenally high, it was remarkably low among the whites although significantly, many of them became ill. But regardless of the label attached to the pandemic, there can be no quibbling about the carnage that ensued.

In February, 1829, the brig *Owhyhee,* commanded by Captain Dominis, arrived from Boston and anchored in the Columbia River. This was the first American trading vessel that had appeared there for fifteen years. It was a long trip from Boston around the Horn, and doubtless there were several stops along the way. We know he paused at the island of Juan Fernandez off the coast of Chile, because he brought some peach trees from there to plant in Oregon. The Indians stoutly maintained that he also brought with him "the fever and ague." A month later the *Convoy,* with Captain Thompson, also from Boston, came to the river.

That spring the water was high and the river overflowed its banks. Furthermore, for the first time ground had been broken in the valley for growing crops. Whether or not these apparently unrelated events were instrumental in providing breeding places for malarial mosquitoes—an easily available source of infection and a vulnerable population—certainly they could have been. In any case the result was incredible.

As Bancroft commented in his *History of the Pacific States of North America,* that summer the outbreak began and within three weeks "fever and ague" swept off the entire Multonomah tribe dwelling on Sauvie Island which lies astride the mouth of the Willamette River. One powerful chief at Fort Vancouver had a thousand warriors prior to that summer, but in one season the disease nearly depopulated the region. The following year was even worse, so that

> the living sufficed not to bury their dead, but fled in terror to the sea-coast, abandoning the dead and dying to the birds and beasts of prey. Every village presented a scene harrowing to the feelings; the canoes were there drawn up upon the beach, the nets extended on the willow-boughs to dry, the very dogs appeared, as ever, watchful, but there was not heard the cheerful sound of the human voice. The green woods, the music of the birds, the busy humming of the insect tribes, the bright summer sky, spoke of life and happiness, while the abode of man was silent as the grave, like it filled with putrid festering corpses.

The Indian population in the Northwest in the four summers during which this epidemic raged was reduced to an estimated fifteen to twenty thousand. Prior to this it had been fully five times as great. In some areas, especially around Fort Vancouver, the mortality reached a staggering 95 per cent. Soon, certainly by 1833 if not earlier, the infection had spread to the California tribes. In general, these were a less resistant group than many of the other natives, and it has been estimated that seventy thousand of them died there of this affliction.

The results of all this must not be underestimated. They were crucial in the development of the Far West. The elimination of some one hundred and fifty thousand natives from the Oregon and California territories could not help but simplify the settlement of those lands by the frontier-pushing Americans. For example, by 1839, an enterprising and energetic individual named John A. Sutter had established himself in the Sacramento Valley. Destiny and empire were breathing on his neck. And by 1846 the ministry in London was well aware that President Polk had an ace in the hole in his diplomatic maneuverings for the Oregon Territory. The Americans had moved into the land they wanted and had no intention of moving out. To try to get them out by combat could be expensive and hazardous. Besides, Oregon was a long way off, whereas a nasty little problem had turned up in Ireland, of all places. Some damnable nuisance was rotting all the potatoes.

The intermittent but nevertheless devastating hammering of disease on the Indian population continued. Sometimes there were tones of sheer tragedy. The most famous example of this occurred during the measles epidemic that struck the Pacific Northwest in 1847. Once again, here was a virus that the natives had never previously encountered, and against which they had no immunity. At the present time measles is frequently looked on as a trivial nuisance that prevents Junior from taking part in the school play or keeps Mother home from the PTA banquet to take care of him. Doubtless the ailment will continue to lose status as modern effective immunizing methods become more widely employed, but as a potential threat for maiming and killing, measles warrants far more than a casual sneer.

The Whitman mission at Waiilatpu, near the present Walla Walla, Washington, had been in existence a little more than ten years when the virulent visitation appeared. The good deeds of the mission had been many, but the sickly Indians, when death struck, soon took a dim view of the white doctor and his medicine. Their own therapeutic armamentarium consisted of sweat baths and cold plunges. The results were promptly, and almost universally, fatal. Unfortunately, for the advance of civilization, Dr. Whitman's therapy was not invariably more favorable. In general, his approach was to treat the disease by more gentle methods. This involved attempts at protection against exposure, the use of warm drinks, the employment of pennyroyal tea, and, in severe cases, purging, bleeding, and catharsis. In other words, he did no harm, and his efforts were relatively innocuous in contrast to the heating and chilling of the sweat bath and the subsequent dive into the river.

Perhaps in this connection a word is in order concerning pennyroyal tea. According to Jacob Bigelow's *Sequel to the Pharmacopoeia of the United States,* published some years prior to this incident, "American pennyroyal is a warm aromatic, possessing a pungent flavour, which is common to many of the labiate plants of other genera. Like them it is heating, carminative and diaphoretic. It is in popular repute as an emmenagogue." An emmenagogue is defined as "a medicine believed to stimulate or restore the normal menstrual function." This, obviously, would be the medication of choice for a measly brave.

But the Indians were dying and the white doctor was not saving them. So the Cayuses in a frenzy of retaliation against they knew not what, massacred Marcus and Narcissa Whitman and twelve others at their tiny mission. So to the Indians at Waiilatpu measles brought death and destruction, and to the Whitmans it brought death and immortality.

As if smallpox, malaria and measles were not enough, there was more trouble afoot. This time, statistically, the white man would suffer far more than the red, but even so, there would be significant fatality among the Indians. Asiatic cholera, which will be dealt with in more detail elsewhere, had ravaged the plains in the years 1832–34 and particularly along the Neosho River, where the Osages alone lost several hundred of their tribe. Actually, this was merely the curtain-raiser. The real trouble from this source began some fifteen years later.

In 1849, brought by the forty-niners as well as the Oregon bound emigrants, cholera again swept along the overland trails, and killed off great numbers of the whites heading for the western Eldorado, and spread promptly to the Indians along the trails. To the Kiowa, dwelling along the northern border of Texas, this was a far more disastrous affliction than smallpox had been a decade before.

Again, also, the Pawnees were slaughtered, so that this large tribe, inhabiting much of what is now Nebraska and Kansas, were reduced to an impotent remnant of their former power. Hunger added to their travail because the herds of buffalo soon began to stay clear of the overland trails. Because of their disease and weakness, the Pawnees could no longer chase the animals into the distant hunting grounds of the Sioux.

There was one further affliction that would lay low the poor Indian, namely tuberculosis. Because of the very nature of the mode of transmission of this disease, it would not deliver its coup de grace for the most part until the tribes were herded together on reservations. Hrdlicka, writing in 1908 says, "[Tuberculosis], which in all probability was extremely rare, if it existed at all, in the prehistoric Indians, and was seldom seen up to a century ago, is gradually becoming everywhere more common, even among the Indians of the Sierras. It attacks especially the adolescents and younger adults. It follows a very rapid course in some individuals and moderately rapid in others, and is nearly always fatal; in a few only it becomes chronic."

According to the National Tuberculosis Asscciation, tuberculosis caused from 26 to 35 per cent of all the deaths occurring among Indians in the decade from 1911 to 1920. During those same years, the examination of more than 600,000 Indians disclosed that 36 per cent of them had tuberculosis.

The result, then, was the destruction of a race. The race was as divergent as any of the others inhabiting the globe. It had a certain shrewdness that enabled it to deal successfully with the climate and the geography to which, over the centuries, it had drifted. It had enough in the way of physical stamina and skill in war to have held out against the conquest for many more years. Its weapons were adequate for the military exigencies of the times, and its warriors demonstrated their ability to adapt themselves to the use of new ones as they came along. They lacked completely any immunity to a whole host of diseases due to microorganisms which the Europeans and Africans brought with them and scattered broadside throughout the New World. Susceptibility to sickness meant weakness in war. Weakness seldom cohabits with justice.

2

The Lion and the Isthmus

Between the reigns of England's two great queens, Elizabeth and Victoria, a little island kingdom became the dominant worldwide empire. To a certain degree the leavening spirit of adventure and the urge to escape religious oppression were motivating factors in this burgeoning, but it is apparent that the major stimulus for this expansion was trade. There were, however, some preliminary considerations to be met. Before Britain could rule more than the most proximal waves, it was necessary for her to control several strategically located points around the globe, not merely for provisioning in the earlier days, and coaling and repair after the advent of steam, but also for purposes of military security. The first of these positions to be taken and held was Gibraltar, but as the years went by, the list grew longer to include such far-flung outposts as Freetown, Capetown, Hong Kong, Singapore, Ceylon, the Falkland Islands, Aden and Suez. Diplomatic maneuvering and military strategy were constantly employed to achieve these objectives. Gold and blood were expended without stint to keep the sun ever high over the British Empire.

It seems strange that a nation so alert to the importance of naval geography, so intent on maintaining its hold on the Mediterranean, the Red Sea, and the Indian Ocean, should have let the Isthmus of Panama slip from its grasp. A close look at history will reveal that this failure was not due to oversight. It was due to considerations poorly under-

43

stood then, and completely disregarded now. The results, nevertheless, were momentous.

Although English mariners ventured into the West Indies within twenty-five years of their discovery by Columbus, these voyages accomplished nothing of significance until 1563 when John Hawkins sold a cargo of slaves to the Spanish. Slavery had been introduced to the area much earlier, but Hawkins gave it new impetus. Peaceful trading, even in human lives, was not to be the order of the day in that part of the world for long. The next act was to be the terror of the Spanish Main and one of the brightest stars of Elizabethan England—Sir Francis Drake.

To understand the motivations of Drake and some of his successors, it is necessary to appreciate what was going on at this time in Spanish America. In 1509 the Spaniards had landed at Cartagena, in what is now Colombia, a couple of hundred miles across the Gulf of Darien from the isthmus, and in the next few years had built a powerful stronghold there. During this same period, fortified towns had been built at Panama on the Pacific coast and on the Atlantic side of the isthmus at Nombre de Dios.

The interests of the Spaniards in the New World were principally metallic. From Peru came gold and silver by ship to Panama. From there, by the year 1530, a broad road had been built, much of it paved, which ran north to Venta Cruces and from there the original route led to Nombre de Dios. Toward the end of the century, because of the poor harbor and because Nombre de Dios was becoming known as the "sepulchre of the Spaniards," this location was practically abandoned. A new city and a new terminus for the trans-isthmian highway was built at Porto Bello about fifteen miles to the west. Along the Gold Road, mule trains carried the precious metals of the New World over which the best blood of the Old was being periodically shed. These ports and this roadway were glittering target areas, and it is to this part of the world that Drake journeyed six times.

His first voyage was as captain of one of Hawkins's ships, and the next two were actually scouting expeditions, but on the fourth trip, in 1572, in a daring but rather ridiculous raid, he attacked the fortified town of Nombre de Dios. Drake entered the town and held it for a matter of hours, but then, wounded himself, he withdrew. With the force at his disposal, there was nothing else he could do. He then based on an offshore island and robbed the mule trains crossing the isthmus, and returned to England in 1573 with silver and gold for ballast.

Much water was to run under Drake's keels before he would again sail to the West Indies, but in September, 1585, with Martin Frobisher as his vice-admiral, he again set forth. This time he tarried at the Cape Verde Islands off the coast of Africa where he undertook an unsuccessful looting sortie. He spent ten days there and burned three towns, but very little of value was carried away. Something unsuspected was taken away, however. Eight days out of Porto Praya, a sailor died of yellow fever. By the time the flotilla arrived at St. Kitts to celebrate Christmas, two hundred of the men were dead and many more invalided. In January, 1586, Drake sacked San Domingo on Hispaniola, and then struck across the Caribbean Sea to the Main. His destination was Cartagena, the most prosperous and commercially the most important city in Spanish America. With the aid of his brilliant land captain, Carleill, he outmaneuvered the Spaniards and captured the town. Drake originally had planned to occupy Cartagena and make it a permanent base from which to destroy the power of Spain in the New World. It was now clear to him that he commanded insufficient strength to achieve this. Instead he spent several weeks conferring with the Spaniards, trying to extort a huge ransom, but while he dallied, the fever again appeared in the fleet.

A general council of land captains was held on February 27 and in the resolution adopted was the statement:

We holder opinion, that with this troope of men which we have presently with us in land-service, being victualled and munitioned, wee may well keepe the towne, albeit that of men able to answere present service, we have not above 700. The residue being some 150 men by reason of their hurts and sicknesse are altogether unable to stand us in any stead: wherefore hereupon the Sea-captaines are likewise to give their resolution, how they will undertake the safetie and service of the Shippes upon the arrival of any Spanish Fleete.

Apparently the "Sea-captaines" were not overconfident either, because as stated later in the same resolution, "And being further advised of the slendernesse of our strengthe, whereunto we be now reduced, as well in respect of the small number of able bodies, as also not a litle in regard of the slacke disposition of the greater part of those which remaine, very many of the better mindes and men being either consumed by death, or weakened by sicknes and hurts." It was then decided to abandon further enterprises and go home.

It had been the original intent that after Cartagena, the fleet would sail to Nombre de Dios and from there a march would be made to Panama and the city looted and destroyed. Drake would then go to Havana, burn it down and build a fortress which would bar the passage of the gold fleet. But the time lost in the Cape Verde Islands, and the fatal infection which had silently crept among the marauders, ruined that ambitious scheme.

Drake sailed home to climax his career by defending England against the Armada, but with his star setting, he started out again in the summer of 1595 with the aging Sir John Hawkins as his vice-admiral and Panama as his objective. There were several diversions along the way, but none of them were profitable. Hawkins died at San Juan, and when Drake finally appeared at the isthmus, having given the defenders ample time to prepare for his coming, he sent an expeditionary force up the old road from Nombre de Dios. Four days later they straggled back, tired, hungry, and defeated. They set fire to Nombre de Dios, shrugged off the failure, raised anchors and set out for

Nicaragua where they had heard the streets were paved with gold. They found no gold, the winds failed them, and for twelve days they beat up and down along the coast. Then the fevers appeared. It was finally decided to sail for Porto Bello, but now officers and men were dying and soon the admiral himself was ill. He had circumnavigated the globe, he had defeated the Armada, and now, off the coast of Darien, he died in a delirium and was buried at sea with no more of a marker for his grave than many a lesser man. With him died the last Elizabethan attempt to seize the isthmus.

A century later the Treaty of Ryswick in 1697 ended an eight-year war with France. It was the signal for British businessmen to expand their trade. Political, religious, and military considerations had combined to put the Scottish merchants in a particularly awkward predicament, and to them the pastures overseas, especially in the Western Hemisphere, appeared enticingly green.

There had been previous attempts at colonization by the Scots at other locations in the New World. Such attempts had been made in Nova Scotia, in New Jersey, and in the Carolinas, but had met with failure. As so often occurs when the occasion demands, a leader emerged, and he was no ordinary man.

William Paterson was born in Dumfrieshire about 1658 and, having acquired a creditable education, left Scotland at an early age and spent several years in the West Indies. He seems to have accumulated a sizeable fortune, and while still in his thirties he returned to London, went into business, and helped to found the Bank of England.

In 1693 the Scottish Parliament passed a general act permitting the formation of joint-stock companies to trade with countries not at war with the British Crown. Such companies were allowed to combine colonizing with their commercial operations. Two years later, with the guiding hand of Paterson apparent in the legislation, an act was passed establishing "The Company for trading from Scot-

land to Africa and all the Indies." The company was capi-
talized at 400,000 pounds, and 1400 Scots put their savings
into the enterprise. There were political ramifications, both
domestic and foreign, that made King William very cool
toward the project, and as a result the government remained officially aloof during the entire affair.

It was Paterson's idea that a colony should be founded
at Darien, on the Isthmus of Panama, which in his own
words was "the key of the Indies and the door of the
world." Paterson fully grasped the importance of the location which would not only furnish a base for operations
against Spain and a storehouse for the West Indian trade,
but also become the trade route to the Orient. In his
communication to the king, Paterson wrote, "Thus, this
door of the seas, and the key of the universe, with anything
of a sort of reasonable management, will of course enable
its proprietors to give laws to both oceans, and to become
arbitrators of the commercial world, without being liable to
the fatigues, expenses, and dangers, or contracting the
guilt and blood, of Alexander and Caesar."

It was a grand scheme, conceived in the grand manner, but there were serious flaws in it. In the first place the
area was obviously Spanish territory although it was not
then occupied by Spaniards. Furthermore, King William,
who was officially at peace with Spain, would perforce take
a dim view of the proceedings. At this time, of course, the
Scots had their own parliament and the situation was
ticklish all around. Aside from the political and diplomatic
ramifications, there were issues of a purely commercial
nature that were handled with less than a strictly realistic
approach. The selection of materials taken along for barter
with the natives was dictated more by the stockholders'
interests than by a genuine appreciation of the sort of
articles likely to be in demand in the tropics. Included in
the cargo were four thousand wigs, which one critic of the
expedition commented sourly could only be used by the
colonists "to mix with their Lyme when they Plaster'd the
Walls of their Houses."

In July, 1698, a fleet of five ships with twelve hundred colonists on board sailed from Leith. After several stops, including a popular one at Madeira, where twenty-seven pipes of wine were taken aboard, they anchored at Darien early in November in a bay which they promptly named Caledonia. Their first act on landing was to build huts to house the many sick on board the ships. It was on this ominous note that the colony of New Edinburgh was begun.

The chosen site appears to have had much to recommend it. There was an excellent harbor, the peninsula was fertile and had good water, and its natural features made it easy to defend. Although the British on Jamaica, reflecting the official attitude, made it apparent that no assistance should be expected from them, provisions were obtained from others whose scruples were not so rigid. The West Indies have always abounded in individuals willing to make a fast piece-of-eight.

In December a report to the homeland disclosed that there had been forty-four deaths on the voyage and thirty-two more in the seven weeks since landing. These were attributed to flux or fever and represented a six percent mortality in six months, including Paterson's wife and the captain of one of the ships.

In February a minor skirmish took place between the Scots and some Spaniards who were scouting the area. One of the ships was sent on a trading expedition but struck a rock near Cartagena and was lost. There were other discouragements, but the greatest was the spectre of death hovering ever closer about the encampment. One of the ship captains later reported, "that their men died and were sick to that height that the liveing were not able to bury the dead; and that they had not six men for guard and sentries; that all manner of distempers, such as head and bellyaches, fevers, fluxes, &c., raged among their men; but all this notwithstanding, the place was very wholesome." Finally, Paterson, the one man with the leadership to inspire the colonists, himself became seriously ill with a fever, and when in June the others decided to abandon the enterprise he was too weak to resist.

The four remaining ships sailed away with the idea of meeting in Boston or Salem, there to sell the rest of their cargoes—the four thousand wigs that had met with sales resistance among the natives, the woolen hats, the heavy stockings and the "Scotch cloath," and the fifteen hundred English Bibles, for which the Caribbean in those days just didn't have the right clientele.

If up to this point the expedition had been unfortunate, it now became a debacle. One of the ships started to sink and was abandoned at sea, some of the survivors landing in Cuba. Another succeeded in getting to Jamaica but was unfit to go farther. The remaining two, the *Caledonia* and the *Unicorn,* both managed to get to New York by August. The captain of the former ship wrote, "In our passage from Caledonia higher our sickness being so universal aboard, and mortality so great that I have hove overboard 105 Corps. The Sickness and Mortality so great that I have burried eleven since I came heire already." The *Unicorn* had no better luck and of the 250 who sailed from Darien only 150 reached New York. Within sixteen months, of the original twelve hundred who sailed with high hopes from Leith, 744 had died. Many of the remainder lost their lives soon after landing in Cuba or Jamaica.

This was not the end of the affair. Communication in those days could go no faster than the hoofs of a horse or the keel of a ship. That summer no one in Scotland realized that the colony had been abandoned. While the *Caledonia* and the *Unicorn* were lying desolately in New York, news arrived that help was on the way from the homeland to Darien. In August two relief vessels appeared at the dreary and deserted site of Caledonia. Shortly after anchoring, the smaller craft burned with all its stores. The men were transferred to the larger ship, and after depositing a dozen volunteers at the barren camp, the remainder sailed to Jamaica. It was late November before the entire relief fleet anchored at Caledonia. In all, some thirteen hundred additional settlers had sailed on this expedition, but already 160 of them had been dropped into the sea. A disheartening scene awaited. The place was deserted, the defenses destroyed, the huts burned. A conference was held and it was voted to land and settle, but before long one of the clergy was writing, "Our sickness did so increase (above 220 at ye same time in fevers and fluxes); and our pitiful rotten provisions were found to be so far exhausted, that we were upon the very point of leaving and losing this colony." Another skirmish occurred with the Spanish on land, and although hailed as a Scottish victory, enemy forces still remained to harass the settlers. At the same time a much more serious threat appeared from seaward. Eleven warships, under command of the Governor of Cartagena, suddenly blocked the harbor entrance. To make matters worse, an accidental fire burned several huts and the situation became grim. Beset by land and by sea, the colonists were now burying up to sixteen of their number each day by virtue of an epidemic. A little over four months after its arrival, the second expeditionary force capitulated to the Spanish and hoisted anchors. The Reverend describes the departure: "As they had been exercised with sore sickness and mortality while in Caledonia, so now when we were at sea, it much increased upon us, and no wonder it was; for the Poor sick men were sadly crouded together, especially aboard the Rising-Sun like so many Hogs in a sty, or sheep in a fold, so that their breath and noisome smell infected and poisoned one another; neither was there anything suitable or comfortable to give the sick and dying; the best was a little spoiled Oat-meal and water. . . ." Of the thirteen hundred who sailed from Scotland on this voyage, at least 920 died and of these only nine were killed by Spaniards.

Following the Treaty of Utrecht in 1713, England was at peace with Spain for a quarter of a century. This was much too long to leave alone a wealthy but feeble competitor, and the English were spoiling for a fight. Walpole, the prime minister, was anxious to avoid war, but he was more

anxious to avoid a turbulent Parliament. Even so, it was
evident that it would take something horrendous to shake
him loose from his position. In the spring of 1739 a member of the House of Commons obliged with the shocking
story of how, three years earlier, a Captain Robert Jenkins
had had his merchant ship confiscated by the Spanish, and
during his remonstrances at the deed, had had an ear
sliced off. The M.P. waved aloft a pathological specimen
purporting to be the amputated pinna for emphasis and
proof. The War of Jenkins' Ear was soon underway.

One of the vociferous members of Parliament most
eager to get the country into the fray was Captain Edward
Vernon, who had had a long career in the navy and who
maintained that given a chance he would take Porto Bello
with six ships. It was generally believed in England at this
time that the capture of Porto Bello and Cartagena would
shatter the power of Spain in the Western Hemisphere.
Cartagena, as we have seen, was ravished by Drake in
1586. More than a hundred years later it had been taken by
the French, but in neither case had there been any attempt
by the conquerors to hold it permanently.

Shortly after the declaration of war, Vernon was commissioned a vice-admiral and sent to the West Indies with
a squadron of nine ships and 3,700 men. With but six of
his ships, he sailed to Porto Bello and put up a furious
cannonade causing the fort at the harbor mouth to surrender, whereupon the city fell without further fighting.

In England the following year, preparations were
made for the much more formidable campaign against
Cartagena. Early July was set as the deadline for sailing,
and Lord Cathcart who was in command was anxious to
avoid delay for he understood the hazards of tropical warfare. His second in command, Brigadier Wentworth, whipped
the raw troops into shape, but someone had neglected
to notify the navy that it might be needed; so the admiral,
who was to escort the transports, had no orders and no
crews. The troops were finally put on board in August, but
for weeks they stayed in port eating up the provisions

intended for the voyage and sickening with scurvy and an infectious fever that raged in the fleet.

At long last the expedition sailed in November, ignoring the fact that time is seldom neutral in war. The transports arrived in the Caribbean in January, 1741. The men were already sickly, more than one hundred of the soldiers were dead, and, most fatal blow of all, Lord Cathcart had died of dysentery on the voyage out.

When the entire force was ultimately assembled in Jamaica, it included several American battalions even worse off than the English. There was not only much sickness among them, but the government in London had overlooked the elementary fact that they would need to be paid and fed. In the first three months, without a shot being fired, of the nine thousand British and Americans, more than six hundred were dead and fifteen hundred were on the sick list.

While the forces were being marshalled the possibility of a preliminary to the main event loomed. A French fleet had been stationed off the coast of Hispaniola for some time, and although England and France were not at war, it seemed risky to take on the Spanish while a potent third force remained in the same waters. The British command resolved to take care of this threat by attacking the French first, but as it happened, the exigency did not arise. Sickness had been so rife among the French sailors that only a sea voyage could restore their health. The fleet had fled the Caribbean miasmas and returned to Brest.

Eventually the expedition was ready. The army was now in command of Brigadier Wentworth who had shown himself to be an excellent drillmaster. Unfortunately, the qualities presently in demand were of a very different order. Vernon, the naval commander, was a man of courage and ability, both fine attributes in such a position; but in war, another element is essential, and that is luck.

By the middle of March, the fleet had anchored off Cartagena and could take stock of the formidable task ahead. The city of Cartagena lay at the end of what

amounted to an inland lake, the entrance to which, from
the sea, was through a narrow passage called Boca Chica,
defended at the time by four forts. To force the Boca Chica
so as to admit the fleet to the harbor was the first objective.
Two of the forts were battered down by part of the naval
squadron on the twentieth of March, and by the twenty-
second a sizeable land force had been put ashore to tackle
one of the others. Wentworth, the training ground general,
was terrified at the thought of being surprised, and literally
stationed so many guards that he could scarcely find
enough men to relieve them. He began to get some tart
suggestions from the navy at this point, but they were
ignored. It was April second before he opened fire on the
fort; and with the help of a cannonade from some of the
men-of-war, the guns of the stronghold were silenced. But
he made no attempt to storm the place two days later. The
exasperated naval high command then urged him to
greater action, adding, "Knowing the climate, we advise you
to pursue more vigorous measures in order to keep your
men from sickness." Goaded by this despatch, Wentworth
ordered the fort to be stormed, whereupon the Spanish fled
almost without firing a shot. The other fortifications were
now abandoned and the entrance of the harbor was open to
the British fleet.

More than a week was wasted transporting the soldiers to the city at the head of the harbor about seven miles
away. During those days the troops broiled, the commanders squabbled, and most significant of all, the mosquitoes
swarmed. Finally the transports arrived and the landing
beach was cleared by shell fire. On the 16th Wentworth
went ashore. He asked for five thousand troops; and since
he was their commander and responsible for land operations, he should have had them without an argument, but
Vernon objected and told him that it would take too long
to debark that many men without their equipment. The
omniscient navy won the debate and fifteen hundred men
were put ashore. In passing it might be noted that practically all the Americans sat out the entire campaign on

board the ships. The high command was dubious about their loyalty and would take no chances with them.

On shore Wentworth with his fifteen hundred men surveyed the situation and found it terrifying. He had but one obstacle between him and Cartagena. This was Fort St. Lazar, and while it was no mean impediment, the probability is that it could have been taken with a rush, but not by the likes of Wentworth who could see himself being ambushed at every rock. So the army encamped and Wentworth demanded the remainder of his five thousand men. These were then sent, and along with them came a nasty note from Vernon pointing out that the Spanish engineers were better than the English and hence delay was Wentworth's worst enemy. The additional time would enable the Spaniards to improve their position and make the task of the assaulting force that much more difficult.

Vernon's contention had more merit than tact, but he was only partly right. Wentworth's worst enemies were not Spaniards. Instead, they were very small, they were airborne and had now been allowed four weeks to make their attack. The general himself probably killed a hundred of them every day with his bare hands, and so did each of his men, but no one thought of them as anything but a nuisance. For the empire they were decisive.

On the 20th of April an assault was made on the north and south sides of Fort St. Lazar. When the soldiers of the king marched out to battle that torrid morning, they left many of their comrades behind. They were lying in camp, dying of yellow fever. The assault was carried out with great courage but little skill, and both were needed. It failed, and of the fifteen hundred English actually engaged, forty-three officers and over six hundred men were killed and wounded. The general did his best to put a good face on the repulse and ordered that a battery be erected to shell Fort St. Lazar on that same evening. It was a fine gesture but it was too late. By this time yellow fever was rampant among the troops, and orders for building batteries would now be canceled by the necessity for digging graves. A council of war was held, and it was decided to abandon the enterprise. A glance at the situation will reveal what impelled that conclusion. Between the morning of April 18th and the night of the 21st, the number of effective troops had dwindled from 6,600 to 3,200. On the 28th, the troops re-embarked, but the transports lay idle in the harbor for one awful week while the death rate constantly mounted. Finally, on the fifth of May it was decided to return to Jamaica. By then the number of men nominally fit for service was down to seventeen hundred, of whom not more than a thousand were in condition to go into combat.

When the ill-starred expedition arrived at Jamaica, the commanders debated subsequent moves and ultimately agreed on Cuba as the next point of attack. But the scourge was not halted by the withdrawal to Jamaica. During the month following the abandonment of Cartagena, there were eleven hundred deaths. The strength of the British sank to fourteen hundred and that of the Americans to thirteen hundred men, and still the ravages of the disease continued. At last the fleet sailed with Santiago de Cuba as its destination and anchored there on August 29. Again there was disagreement between the energetic admiral and the reluctant general as to the conduct of the campaign. While the troops lay idle in their camp and the rainy season drew to a close, the sickness increased rather than abated. By the middle of November it was difficult to find enough men to relieve the guards, and in another two weeks there were fewer than three hundred privates fit for duty. Once more the campaign was abandoned and the weary ships returned to Jamaica.

In February, 1742, a reinforcement of three thousand men came from England. They arrived in good health but began to sicken almost at once. While the commanders discussed new projects, the soldiers died at the rate of a hundred a week. Finally a decision was reached. This time they would strike once more against the mainland, and it would be at the same point on the isthmus where Vernon had had his initial triumph a year and a half before. Again the fleet put to sea and headed for Porto Bello. The weather did not favor the invaders, and the crossing took nineteen days; and with them rode the pestilence. During that voyage, ninety-eight bodies from one regiment alone were flung into the turbulent sea.

Vernon landed and reoccupied Porto Bello as the point from which the march across the isthmus to the city of Panama was to begin. The admiral was not to have his second victory, however. The roster of the troops by now showed that nearly a thousand were sick or dead. There was nothing they could do but withdraw. By the time they had returned, they discovered that five hundred more of the sick that had been left behind in Jamaica were now dead. Of the original regiments that had sailed with Cathcart, nine men in every ten had perished.

The next attempt of the British to capture a foothold on the isthmus took place during the American Revolution. To His Majesty's Government the suppression of the colonial revolt was only one objective in what, from its point of view, was a global war. When the Spanish entered the engagement along with the French, the war theater became enlarged. The Caribbean area, during the early years of the conflict, had been a source of great irritation to the ministry in London. Partly due to frank treachery by some of the English colonials, partly due to smuggling in which many nationalities, especially the Dutch, were involved, the West Indies had become a major source of supply for the rebellious colonies. With Spain an avowed belligerent, it now became possible for the Royal Navy to move with greater freedom in these parlous waters.

At this time General John Dalling, governor of Jamaica, submitted to the British government a plan for a military and naval expedition to Nicaragua. During the previous year, Manuel Galisteo had been sent to investigate for the King of Spain the possibilities of a canal through Nicaragua. British agents from Belize had managed to accompany the party in a private capacity; and whereas Galisteo had sent his government an unfavorable report, the British had informed London that the project appeared entirely feasible. When Dalling's recommendation arrived, therefore, it was promptly approved by the British cabinet, and the plan was executed.

The idea was to capture and occupy the river and castle of St. Juan and the Lake of Nicaragua with the cities on both Atlantic and Pacific coasts. This would effectively cut communication between the northern and southern Spanish territories. It would do something else. It would put the British lion astride the isthmus at the only location considered at that time to be practicable for a canal.

St. John's River flows from Lake Nicaragua ninety-six miles through rugged country to the Atlantic. The initial expedition, led by Colonel Polson, sailed from Jamaica on March 4, 1780. The convoy was commanded by an energetic and inspiring young naval officer who landed the troops safely at St. John's Harbor and then volunteered to accompany Polson up the river with the small boats and some of his sailors. It was sixty-four miles upstream from the harbor to the fort of St. Juan and it took a week, struggling against the shoals and the rapids in the stifling heat, to reach that destination. Sickness was now prevalent among the men; but with the untiring energy of two officers, the chief engineer and the naval officer who laid many of the guns with their own hands, the little force succeeded in besieging the castle and cutting off its supply of water until it capitulated. "Thus," crowed Gov. Dalling a bit prematurely, "the door to the South Seas is burst open."

By this time the naval officer was seriously ill. It was imperative that he be evacuated, so he was sent downriver to the harbor. For here was not a man destined to be buried in a mangrove swamp or to be thrown into the ocean with a round-shot at his heels. Instead he would someday lie under the great dome of St. Paul's Cathedral in London, where a grateful nation would place him. For this was Nelson, and over the distant horizon, far beyond the chills and sweats of Nicaragua, were waiting Aboukir Bay and Trafalgar.

It was still thirty-two miles to the lake, and the present force was too feeble to garrison what it held. Reinforcements were sent from Jamaica under Brigadier General Stephen Kemble who was to take over command of the expedition. Kemble was an American, born in New Jersey, and had been a commissioned officer in His Majesty's Army since 1757. He kept a journal of the campaign, and his orders have also been preserved. From these sources may be obtained an excellent picture of what he had to face.

On April 10, 1780, he sailed from Jamaica and arrived at St. John's Harbor ten days later. Some time was spent in organizing the installation at the river's mouth, and then he started for the castle. On his way up the river he wrote in his journal, "Wednesday, May 10th . . . proceeded about ten miles through a continued heavy Rain; encamped upon a sandy point about 3 o'clock; made a large fire and dried our moist Blankets and Clothes: but we were pestered with such numbers of Mosquitoes that we could take no rest." He arrived at the castle on May 15th, and shortly thereafter is the somewhat wistful entry, "From my arrival gave every direction for the Preservation or Provision, Stores, etc.; but have no one to put it in Execution, all being Sick."

It would be more than a hundred years before the overwhelming importance of mosquitoes would be realized, but Kemble did what he could to improve the sanitation of the post. A general order was issued on 21st May. "It is Brig. Gen. Kemble's positive Orders that all men who Die are buried at least Sixty Yards beyond the Magazine Tent, and that the People employed in making the Grave are particularly careful that it is not less than four feet deep." And on the following day, "Necessary Places being made in front of the Encampment, No Soldier or other person whatever to Ease himself anywhere else. And as nothing Contributes more to the preservation of health than Cleanliness, Such as are found to disobey this Order may depend upon being Severely punished." But it was not enough for we read in the Journal, "Wednesday, May 24th. Nothing Extraordinary, but the increase of our Sick."

Two days later he was sick himself, and by June first, "Not capable, from my extreme illness, of doing any business. Dr. Welche's fatigue has brought a Fever on him." The entries continue. On June 30th, "The Mortality and great Sickness of the Soldiery give me much uneasiness; the Officers also very low for want of proper Nourishment."

In spite of all this the campaign went on and an attempt was made to capture the upper fort where the river emerged from the lake. The feeble assault failed, and from then on the situation rapidly deteriorated. By this time about fourteen hundred men had been sent to Nicaragua; but at the end of September only 320 of them, blacks and whites, were left alive, while of these not one-half were fit for duty. Orders from Dalling were eventually received, whereupon the castle was blown up, and Nicaragua was evacuated.

This should have been enough, but there was to be one more abortive attempt to take the isthmus, the frailest of them all, in the nineteenth century.

One day in the fall of 1822 a young surgeon was whiling away his time in London, waiting for a ship to take him to a new appointment in Bengal. He occupied himself most profitably during the interval by attending the lectures at Guy's Hospital given by Sir Astley Cooper, the leading surgeon of his day. A notice on the bulletin board outside the lecture hall caught the young man's eye. There was an opening for a well-qualified surgeon to accompany a party of settlers to Poyais on the Mosquito Shore of Honduras. "The Territory of Poyais . . . is situated on the mountainous side of the Bay of Honduras. . . . The Climate is remarkably healthy, and agrees admirably with the constitution of Europeans." So read the rhapsodic circular on the Poyais Land Office published November 1, 1822.

At the time there was considerable discussion in the London press about this venture, some insisting that the entire project was mere "loan jobbery" and "land jobbery" to victimize the gullible; and others maintaining that the strip of territory involved with its access through the San Juan River to Lake Nicaragua was of such prospective value to Great Britain as a canal route that the government should seriously consider its acquisition. Whatever the government's serious consideration may have been, there was no attempt to impede the enterprise, and at least several functionaries cooperated.

To young Dr. James Douglas the proposition sounded more appealing than India. He applied for the job, was accepted and on November 22nd embarked at Gravesend with the commandant, two other officials and seventy-three settlers, including some women and children. They arrived at their destination, the mouth of the Black River on the Mosquito Shore, in February, but looked in vain for the buildings they had been told would be there. Later they found the ruins of some of these entirely engulfed by the tropical forest, but for now living space and living quarters had to be hacked out of the jungle.

In March, several cases of bilious fever appeared. By that time supplies were short—even the rum was gone— and Dr. Douglas noted in his journal, "I had nothing but my lancets and a phial of tartar emetic." At the end of the month he had ten cases of fever "of more than ordinary intensity."

At this point the situation was enlivened in the frail little colony by the arrival of 160 new settlers who brought with them scarcely enough provisions to get them ashore. By mid-April the rains increased, there were more fevers, and one man died. Ten days later, out of a colony now numbering 220 (there had been a few deserters and one suicide), all were sick except nine. The situation continued to worsen. In May a small schooner arrived and removed fifty-seven of the sick to Belize; and in June the remainder of the colonists, including Dr. Douglas, himself desperately ill, were evacuated. The Poyais Settlement, having accomplished nothing except to add to the European saga of tropical misery, had lasted a scant five months.

There is no satisfactory way, at this date, to make an accurate modern diagnosis of many of the ailments prevalent centuries ago. Just as kingdoms and races flourish and fade, so do diseases. Organisms may become attenuated, or conditions favorable to their propagation may disappear, or the victim may develop an immunity. The disease in question either vanishes or only occurs in mild form and occasional instance.

There can be no doubt that the prevalent infection at Cartagena, and in many other locations in the Caribbean, was yellow fever. Malaria was presumably the villain in Honduras and definitely brought about the downfall of the Nicaragua sortie. The "ague" occurring on alternate days, the relapses that invariably developed upon return to duty, and the relief of Kemble's own symptoms when "the bark" eventually became available, all incriminate malaria. The fluxes could have been any of the enteric fevers, such as typhoid or bacillary dysentery or related infections, or there may well have been rampant at the time some microbial agents that have since disappeared.

Here, then, is a story extending over a period of 250 years. Nombre de Dios, Darien, Cartagena, Porto Bello, Nicaragua, the Mosquito Coast, the high seas and the sultry shallows—these places meant suffering, sorrow and death to thousands of persons, many of whom merely had the misfortune to wander out on a dark London street when a press gang swept by. These thousands are all but forgotten, and they are forgotten because they failed. No nation's historians dwell for long over its failures. And yet these men did not fail due to lack of courage, for this they possessed beyond measure. Their training, their equipment, and their leadership were equal to that of their brothers who were at the same time winning victories in other parts of the world. They failed because of an enemy they could not battle, and which neither they nor their wiser contemporaries even realized existed. The British lion was frustrated in his determined attempt to control the Panamanian isthmus, not by broadswords and cutlasses, not by fortresses and fascines, not by cannon and muskets, but by bacteria and viruses and mosquitoes and flies.

3

The Maple Leaf Forever

KING WILLIAM'S WAR

With ambitious European nations colonizing and claiming for themselves large sections of the rich areas of the New World, it was only natural that there should be sanguinary and protracted conflict over the possession of these dominions. Spain was a special problem, and she confined her interests primarily to the warmer regions. The Dutch, also, hardly qualified as a major contender. The principal struggle for North America was destined to be between England and France.

Off and on over a period of many years, the early colonists in what is now the eastern half of the United States and Canada snarled at each other and occasionally came to grips. There were skirmishes and sometimes devastating raids, but much more of the attentions of both nationalities, in the early days, were occupied with the hazards of the wilderness, the climate, and the Indians. The latter were sometimes an ally of one or the other, but more often an enemy of both.

Toward the end of the seventeenth century, events on both sides of the Atlantic caused a turbulent situation to erupt into open war. In 1685 the French in Canada were in serious trouble with the Iroquois. Louis XIV was determined to control the situation, and so, typical of administrative procedure before and since, he selected a new governor to clear up the matter. In June the governor, Denonville, sailed from France, but the voyage was inauspicious.

So poorly equipped were his ships that a quarter of the six hundred soldiers embarking with him died of fever and scurvy during the crossing. When the wretched survivors finally landed at Quebec, the nuns of the Hôtel Dieu were utterly overwhelmed with the problem of caring for the multitude of sick.

The new governor was beset with difficulties requiring far more in the way of troops and money than had been made available to him. His enemies fully appreciated Denonville's weaknesses. The Indians were both insolent and demanding. At the same time the English threatened from two directions, Hudson's Bay and New England. As matters worsened, the situation again, from the viewpoint of Paris, demanded another change of leadership, and the hapless Denonville was recalled.

The struggle that began started not solely because of the unsettled state of affairs on this continent. The explosion might have been set off here by any of the various skirmishes and insults that had taken place over the previous unsettled years, but now the torch was aflame as well in Europe. It was at this point that the revolution occurred in England, and James II, the ally of France, was driven from his kingdom, while William of Orange crossed the North Sea to seize the vacant throne.

In North America the Grand Monarch was facing a grim predicament. The Iroquois alone had brought the French colony to the brink of ruin, and now the savages would be abetted by the irritating British colonies to the south, relatively rich and populous, compared to the depleted settlements of Canada. Unquestionably, Louis XIV was rapidly becoming disenchanted with his empire in North America. It had not prospered as he had been told it would. Furthermore the mortality in this distant and expansive wilderness was distressingly high. He determined, however, to make one more major attempt to salvage this hideous situation, but to do so called for strong measures. Some years earlier the Count Frontenac had been recalled from these same northern settlements, if not in disgrace at least under a cloud. But he, of all Frenchmen, was adored by the colonists and respected by the Indians. This was not the time for the indulgence of royal pride. In October, 1689, Frontenac sailed from France for his second term as governor.

When Frontenac sailed from France the grand strategy called for a prompt conquest of the colonies of upper New York, considered as ripe for the plucking at that moment. However, by the time he arrived at Quebec he realized that both the Iroquois and the English were fully alerted to the new danger and the projected expedition must be abandoned. He was three months too late.

Even so, things began happening rapidly in the spring of 1690. Frontenac felt that his major opponent should be the English rather than the Indians, recognizing that the former represented the greater threat to the ultimate future of France. It was against the colonists, therefore, that he mounted his principal offensive. His immediate plan was to organize three war parties of select men, skilled in winter travel overland; one at Montreal, one at Three Rivers and one at Quebec. The first expedition was intended to strike at Albany, but because of the bitter weather the attack was made on Schenectady, the farthest outpost of the colony of New York, then inhabited by Dutch. There, except for a handful of escapees, the entire village was massacred or taken prisoner. From Three Rivers a party set out in the dead of winter for the New Hampshire settlements and sacked Salmon Falls and the surrounding sparsely settled area, and then joined up with the third band of French and Indians on its way from Quebec to attack the forts on the coast of Maine. One of their objectives was on Casco Bay, a settlement located in what is now Portland. Its capture, because of the strategic importance of this outpost, caused great alarm in Massachusetts.

While all this was going on the opposition was not idle. Serious commercial problems had been plaguing the New England seacoast colonies for some years. During the entire colonial period, the wealth of coastal New England would literally come from the sea, either as a source of fish, or as a means of transport of slaves, timber, molasses, rum, or the luxuries of the Orient. Agriculture would scarcely support a meager inland population, whereas manufacturing was nonexistent in the early years due to lack of equipment and skill and in later times to the doctrinaire attitude of the British.

The economic foundation of colonial New England was strictly maritime. The French naturally were jealous of the New England seaborne trade and had taken some pains to interfere with its success. Port Royal on Annapolis Harbor on the Bay of Fundy provided a convenient harborage for French cruisers that were particularly active in harassing Massachusetts shipping in recent years. In April a vessel was sent to England bearing urgent messages warning of the exposed state of the colony and pleading for the prompt reduction of Canada. Requests were made for arms, ammunition, and a squadron of frigates to attack the French by sea, whilst colonial forces would invade the enemy territory by land. Unfortunately for the colonial cause, King William, at this juncture, had other vexations on his royal mind. He was busy fighting James in Ireland, and it might be noted in passing that the flux and fever in his army were causing him fully as much concern as either the Irish or his father-in-law. In any case, he sent no help, but even worse, no reply at all arrived in Massachusetts for many months.

The most colorful and probably the most capable man in the colony of Massachusetts at the time was Sir William Phips, a local boy who had made good in divers ways. He had started out as a ship's carpenter, had married well, and had retrieved a Spanish treasure ship in the Caribbean; and he was an obvious leader of men. He was promptly appointed to the command. Phips sailed from Hull—then called Nantasket—on the twenty-eighth of April, found the fort at Port Royal in no condition to withstand a siege, demanded and received its surrender and returned to Boston in triumph on the thirtieth of May.

When Phips arrived home he immediately discovered there was much more work to be done. During his absence a congress of delegates from the various English colonies in the Northeast had been held in New York. It had been agreed that a joint attack should be mounted against Canada. New York was to furnish several hundred men and the New England colonies the remainder.

These were to rendezvous at Albany and march on Montreal. While that stronghold was thus assailed by land, Massachusetts and the other New England colonies were to attack Quebec by sea, establishing a pincers strategy that would be invoked many times in the coming years. After much haggling it was decided that Fitz-John Winthrop of Connecticut should be placed in command of the land forces and Robert Livingston of New York would be his lieutenant.

In Boston there was great activity. The provisional government of Massachusetts accepted the responsibility and borrowed money, called for volunteers, pressed men when the volunteers were not eagerly forthcoming, chose its new hero, Phips, as commander, and gave John Walley of Barnstable the unenviable position of second-in-command.

About the middle of July all preparations were reported as ready for the expedition, but Phips delayed embarkation in the hope that some reply to the request for aid might be received. None was forthcoming, and he finally sailed on the ninth of August. There were between thirty and forty vessels, great and small, and the fleet, including sailors, carried 2,200 men with provisions for four months but insufficient ammunition and no pilot for the St. Lawrence.

At this point it might be well to note what was happening to the land forces. According to the plan settled on at the New York conference, two thousand were expected to march by Lake Champlain and attack Montreal, at the same time that the forces by sea should be before Quebec.

It didn't work out as planned. Having received a commission from Governor Treat of Connecticut "to command the forces designed against Canada," Winthrop set out from Hartford accompanied by Livingston. After a week's march "through the difficult and almost impassable parts of the wilderness," the Connecticut general reached Kinderhook, where some of the Albany officers hastened to meet him. On reaching Albany, Winthrop made Livingston's house his headquarters and "found the design against Canada poorly contrived and little prosecuted, all things confused, and in no readiness or posture for marching."

That was only the beginning. He had many more problems. The militia were assembling but their strength was less than he had been promised. One reason was that not until after the New York conclave had it been fully realized in Massachusetts Bay and Plymouth the extent of the disaster suffered in Maine the previous winter at the hands of Frontenac's raiders. Thereupon these colonies decided to use their levies to protect their own frontiers rather than sacrifice them on the uncertainties of foreign service. Winthrop surveyed what was left. Smallpox was epidemic in Albany that summer, and there already had been inroads on his forces. To add to his miseries, dysentery had reared its ugly aspect.

Despite all this, the little army began its march to Lake Champlain with motley collections of Mohawk, Oneida, and Mohegan allies. Their first destination was to be Wood Creek, near the head of the lake, from whence they planned to embark for the north. During the march Major General Winthrop made an ominous entry in his diary on the 28th of July, noting that there was "an increase of the small pox in the army, many being dead in the several countries."

When the sickly band arrived at Wood Creek a council of war was held. The savages advised the army to advance immediately to Isle La Motte, at the northern end of the lake, where the western Iroquois were to join and reinforce the expedition. But disastrous news soon came that the

Senecas, on whom the provincials largely depended for support, were suffering from epidemic smallpox and "that the Great God had stopt their way." In spite of this dismaying intelligence, an attempt would be made to traverse the length of the lake—the gateway to the heart of Canada—and to that end boats were to be built. This produced problems, too. In this locality birch was not available in quantity, and so an attempt was made to build canoes of elm bark. This was a failure. If it is too late in the season, elm bark will not peel and so again the expedition was frustrated. But at this point the ultimate catastrophe occurred. Suddenly smallpox broke out with renewed fury. Another council of war was held, and at this meeting, "it was thought most advisable to return with the army."

The decision was fateful. Montreal was no longer threatened. Disheartened by circumstances he could not control, Winthrop led his little army back, "many of the soldiers being sick and lame," and in a few days encamped it at Greenbush, opposite Albany. One arm of the pincers was shattered. Phips would have to conquer Canada alone.

Phips was to find that the campaign against Quebec was not going to be the pushover that the capture of the relatively miniature fortress of Port Royal had been. The commander essayed the tactics that had been so successful at Port Royal and demanded the surrender of Quebec. This time he simply did not have the cards or the terrified opponent, and the French called his bluff. Frontenac had received the information some time earlier that Winthrop was not coming down the lake to attack Montreal, and so the French governor, knowing that that city was in no danger, had brought from there a sizeable contingent to aid in the defense of Quebec. It was at this point that Frontenac scornfully told the envoy of the New Englander that he would answer him only by the mouths of his cannon.

After considerable delay the colonists finally arranged

a plan of attack, and the militia, under Walley, landed at Beauport, below Quebec. The landing was difficult, the water was low, and the boats grounded before reaching the landing place. Walley's journal eloquently describes the situation, "Oct. 8. The cold of the night and our souldiers not having opportunity to dry themselves, gott what refreshment they could . . . being more and more sensible of the enemies strength, and our own men, many, growing sick and unfitt for service." Phips, with his feeble cannon in the fleet, blasted futilely away at the cliffs of Quebec while Walley lay in his frigid camp—his men wet, shivering with cold, famished, and sickening with smallpox. Several minor skirmishes occurred in the next few days, but it soon became apparent that this was a thoroughly useless enterprise. The men were re-embarked and the New Englanders withdrew.

There is an extremely ironic overtone to the timing of Phips's attack. The French themselves admit that if he had arrived a week earlier, which he could easily have done, there were then only two hundred regular troops in Quebec. The city was exposed on every side and could have been taken without striking a blow. On the other hand, if he had held out for one more week, the town might have surrendered, because the sudden and unexpected influx of troops had caused such a drastic drain on the food supply of the garrison that it was nearing starvation just as the last sail of the attacking fleet was disappearing beyond the Isle d'Orleans.

Phips arrived crestfallen at Boston on November 19, 1690, having lost more than two hundred of his men from smallpox and fever. Chevalier de Callieres refers to the dispersion of Winthrop's army and the defeat of Phips in his communication to M. de Seigneley in 1690, "Small pox broke out among their land forces and destroyed from four to five hundred men on the march. This obliged them to return, and we have been sufficiently fortunate to drive their fleet from before Quebec."

After the second and humiliating return of Phips as a military leader to Boston, there were many raids in the colonies involving the Indians, the French, and the English. Distressing though they may have been, they had little effect on the progress of the war. Ultimately the royal court came to believe that genuine advantage would accrue to the crown if a full-scale attack on Canada were to be mounted. In 1692, London resolved on an expedition for the following year. This was to be an ambitious undertaking. During the winter a considerable strength of ships and men under Admiral Sir Francis Wheeler would sail to the West Indies, reduce the French stronghold of Martinico, and having taken care of that detail proceed to Boston by the first of June. The furtherance of the scheme called for a sizeable body of Massachusetts forces under the command of Sir William Phips to be then taken aboard and the whole force would sail to the St. Lawrence. The fall of Quebec would then require only a minor military exercise.

The plan was excellent. There were a few things preventing its auspicious execution. The least of these was that no one in New England had heard anything of this magnificent design until Admiral Wheeler arrived in the port of Boston on the eleventh of June. By this time the sailors were off to the fishing grounds. Although conceivably a land army might have been recruited, such would have been of scant aid. While in the West Indies the Admiral's powerful fleet had been attacked by a devastating airborne armada of mosquitoes. By the time Wheeler arrived in Boston he had buried 1,300 out of 2,100 sailors and 1,800 of 2,400 soldiers. This may have represented the first outbreak of yellow fever ever to occur in North America. It is certainly possible, biologically, for the yellow fever mosquito to survive the passage from the West Indies to Boston in the summer. The packed masses of British soldiers and sailors would easily provide an ample supply of human hosts to keep the virus happy and prolific during the voyage. The effect in Boston itself was disastrous as Cotton Mather makes clear in his diary. "In the month of

*July** a most pestilential Feaver, was brought among us by the Fleet coming into our Harbour from the West-Indies. It was a Distemper, which in less than a Week's time usually carried off my Neighbours, with very direful Symptoms, of turning *Yellow,* vomiting and bleeding every day and so Dying; tho' for diverse Dayes after the first Decumbiture, the Disease did but as it were play with the Sick." For obvious reasons there was no expedition against Quebec in 1693. Things were relatively quiet also during 1694 and as to the year after that, Hutchinson explains why there was again a military interlude. "The year 1695 passed away, with less molestation from the enemy, than any year since 1688 . . . A mortal sickness prevailed among the Indians, and the French found it impractical to send them out in parties upon our frontiers."

The French in Canada, too, were demanding help from the homeland. Finally after many delays the Marquis de Nesmond, in May, 1697, with a powerful squadron of fifteen ships, sailed for Newfoundland with orders to defeat an English fleet loaded with salt for the fisheries and supposed to be in that neighborhood. The Marquis was then ordered to proceed to the Penobscot where he would be joined by a contingent of Abenaki warriors and fifteen hundred troops from Canada. The whole united force would then fall upon Boston. The plan of attack was designed with considerable care and took advantage of the seasonal fact that much of the seafaring manpower would be absent from Massachusetts harvesting fish. Boston would be destroyed, and the North Shore as far as Portsmouth would be ravished. Again, this time for the French, things went wrong. Headwinds delayed the fleet and provisions began to run short. Apparently scurvy appeared, and this disheartened the commanders to the point that the assault was abandoned. Cotton Mather, in a November 1697 entry in his diary, has this to say: "A formidable

* Hutchinson says the fleet arrived June eleventh. Perhaps Mather means that the epidemic had really become established by the following month.

Squadron of about fifteen French Men of War, were coming to this Town, and would, no doubt, have laid it very
desolate: but when they were a little Way off, the *Angel of
the Lord went forth,* and smote 'em with such a wasting
Sickness, that the Loss of their Men by it, enfeebled 'em so
as to make 'em desert the Enterprise."

There was no further consequential action during the
war, and the Peace of Ryswick was proclaimed in Boston
the following month.

QUEEN ANNE'S WAR

Less than five years passed before France and England were once again at each other's throats. Again, as it
would so often, the excuse for conflict devolved around the
occupancy of European thrones. In North America the
change in the situation was minimal. The Indians, who
supported the French, had scarcely left the warpath during the supposedly peaceful interval and were now pad-
ding along familiar trails with enthusiastic royal support
from thousands of miles away. The immediate result was a
series of vicious border raids in which many stalwart settlers were killed and women and children carried off as
captives.

The military problem facing the colonists was grim.
Reprisals for raids such as they were currently suffering
were nearly impossible. An example was the attack in
February, 1704, on Deerfield, Massachusetts, a village of
no military or political importance. There were others of a
similar nature. Bands of marauders, usually composed of
both French and Indians, swooped down from the north,
struck in the night, pillaged and burned and then vanished
like smoke in a breeze. To try to combat such a threat by
chasing down a handful of Indians to their camps was
useless. The only practical approach was to strike at the
heart of the enterprise.

Port Royal, once again in French hands, was the first
objective of the English. It was a noble objective. The

flotilla arrived at Port Royal on the 10th of August, 1707, but the men were in poor condition either to attack or sustain a siege. "There is a considerable number of them visited with violent fluxes . . . others taken with mighty swellings in their throats . . . in a short time, there will not be well enough to carry off the sick. . . ." After ten days of this sort of misery the attackers withdrew.

The next significant move in this conflict was on the part of an ambitious colonist named Samuel Vetch, who was sent to England to ask for help in the reduction of Canada. The court was in a good mood, granted all that Vetch requested, and he sailed gleefully for home in March, 1709. Governor Dudley was advised that the French were to be subdued not only in Canada and Acadia, but in Newfoundland as well. A squadron of ships would be in Boston Harbor by the middle of May. Five regiments of regulars were to be sent from England to be joined by twelve hundred men to be raised in Massachusetts and Rhode Island. With this force Quebec was to be attacked. At the same time fifteen hundred men raised from New York, New Jersey, Pennsylvania, and Connecticut were to make the now familiar journey by Lake Champlain and the rivers and take Montreal. Canada would be English territory.

This time the land and fresh water expedition was commanded by Colonel Francis Nicholson, recently lieutenant-governor of New York, who moved his force from Albany up the Hudson and thence overland to Wood Creek where a fort was built. Flat boats and canoes were constructed, supplies were brought in and all was in readiness to embark for Montreal and glory. One thing delayed them. They must wait for word that the British fleet had arrived in Boston. It was a long wait.

It was a hot summer. Nicholson's choice of a campsite was in a swampy area. There were flies and there were mosquitoes. Soon there was dysentery—sudden, violent and frequently fatal. One account maintains that the Iroquois had an etiologic role in the spread of the disease.

Undoubtedly this tribe had shrewdly determined that it would be very much to their own self-interest to see to it that neither the English nor the French ever became powerful enough to eliminate the other. From their observation, Nicholson had sufficient force to capture Montreal. In order to prevent this the Indians supposedly polluted the water of Wood Creek, upstream from the encampment, by throwing skins and dead animals into it. Whether or not Indian familiarity with public health measures combined with treachery played a part in this epidemic, the results were disastrous. It would be a long time before the concept of filtering or chlorinating water would become a part of military hygiene; but the soldiers "died as if they had been poisoned." A party of French who visited the spot later in the autumn stated that judging by the graves, at least a thousand must have been buried there.

The ultimate act of sabotage of the entire expedition had already been performed in London. The fleet, expected to arrive in Boston in May, had sailed instead to settle some trivial Iberian issue in Portugal. There was no naval force for New England.

In December, 1709, Nicholson sailed for England to solicit the aid of the crown against Canada. His reception was favorable, and he returned in the spring commissioned to command an enterprise against Port Royal with Vetch as adjutant-general. On the 18th of September, a fleet of thirty-six sail, a regiment of marines and four regiments of colonials raised in New England finally set forth and arrived at their destination six days later. After the exchange of a few shots and many messages, the fort surrendered, a garrison was left and the remainder returned to Boston late in October.

Nicholson commuted to London again that fall, and again his voyage was productive. In June, 1711, much to the amazement of nearly everyone, Admiral Sir Hovenden Walker arrived at Boston with a sizeable fleet and army to settle the matter of Canada once and for all. Nicholson scurried back to Albany at the end of July to take charge of another Montreal-bound contingent, and Walker sailed for the St. Lawrence on the same day with more than seventy ships and nearly twelve thousand men. In the great gaping mouth of the St. Lawrence, the fleet ran into a storm and several ships foundered on a reef. The loss, when it was counted up, consisted of ten vessels, more than nine hundred lives and Walker's nerve. The fleet withdrew and the expedition was abandoned. When the news of Walker on the rocks reached Nicholson, tenting on the old campsite at Wood Creek, he tore off his wig, threw it on the ground in frustration and rage, stamped on it, delivered himself of a few unrecorded phrases and trudged back to Albany.

It is quite possible that there was one positive result from "Shipwreck" Walker's otherwise disastrous expedition. Port Royal, from now on to be known as Annapolis Royal, had been garrisoned following its capture the year before by a few hundred colonial militia. During the spring of 1711, "a pestilence," the nature of which is obscure, struck the garrison, and the mortality was so great that the survivors were afraid even of the ordinarily peaceful Acadians alone. The French, who were well aware of the situation, had raised troops who were about to set out for Nova Scotia and the inevitable recapture of the port. At this point news arrived that Walker was on his way and so the French retained their troops for the defense of Canada. This time, when peace came again, England held on to Acadia, but the French kept valuable Cape Breton; and on the southeastern part of that island, they would build Louisbourg, soon to become recognized as the strongest fortress in the New World.

WAR OF THE AUSTRIAN SUCCESSION

In 1745 the wintry streets of Boston were slippery, just as they are now. One January day of that year a member of the General Court, while hurrying to attend a special session of that august body, fell and broke his leg. It was a momentous fracture. The injured man, if present at the assembly, would have opposed a measure that passed by a single vote. By this meager margin the decision was reached whereby Massachusetts, unaided by the king, and with sparse help from a few other colonies, would launch an attack against the most formidable fortress in the Western Hemisphere.

Some years earlier England had gone to war with Spain, in part at least to preserve the inalienable right of British mariners to wear two ears. It was inevitable, with these nations engaged, that the French would soon become embroiled. The government in London was too preoccupied with events close to home to inform their colonies of any change in diplomatic status. But the French were less diffident about notifying their North American outposts. As soon as the news of declaration of war arrived in May, 1744, immediate preparations were made by the French at Louisbourg to attack the nearest British settlement, a fishing station at Canso on a barren island in Nova Scotia some fifty miles away. This establishment was burned to the ground; and although it was a poor place with only some 150 wooden buildings, it was important to the New England fishery, and its loss created much anguish in Massachusetts.

The sole British military post in the entire area was Annapolis, the former Port Royal, which since its capture a quarter century before had become a lonely, rundown station with only a few hundred defenders surrounded by French inhabitants and therefore in constant danger. Nova Scotia, however, represented New England's principal outpost of defense in the north against the ravaging of its coastal towns by a French fleet.

It was under such circumstances that an attack on Louisbourg appeared necessary, and perhaps feasible, to the New England colonies, and especially to Massachusetts. At the moment there was almost no one in the colonies with anything that might be considered worthwhile military experience, so Governor Shirley drew up a

plan of attack and appointed William Pepperrell to the
command. One commentator of the time said that the
expedition had a lawyer for contriver, a merchant for
general, and farmers, fishermen, and mechanics for soldiers. On Sunday, the 24th of March, 1745, the fleet,
consisting of about ninety transports, escorted by provincial cruisers and with about four thousand untrained men
aboard, sailed from Nantasket Roads.

The first difficulty to be encountered by the newly
designated combatants is a situation familiar to the present
day. According to one diarist:

> 27 Wednesday this day our Vessel was A Very Hospital, wee were
> all Sick, in a Greater or lesser Degree. Wee Sail'd a good pace all
> Day, Towards Night, the Wind Began to rise, it also Grew foggy
> and Something rainy. So That wee Could not be Upon Deck, as
> the Night before—But was Shut down in the hold; and a Long,
> Dark and Tedious night wee had, Such a one as I Never See
> before: Wee was also Much Crouded, even So as to Lay, one on
> Another. Sick etc. My Friends, you can Scarsely think What
> Distress wee were in.

> Thursday 28 Our disstress Encreas'd, inasmuch as our Sickness,
> not only Continued, but the weather Grew, Thicker and more
> Stormy. And our Captain Upon whom (Under God) was our
> dependence Began to Drink too hard. As the Storm Encreas'd (As
> is too frequently the Manner of Seamen) So that he was
> Altogether Uncapable to manage the Vessel. . . .

The same writer gives us an eloquent word picture of
the infantry training to which this colonial army was subjected. The fleet gathered at Canso, destroyed—as previously noted—but not occupied by the French.

"Thursday (April . . . New Hampshire Soldiers were
all Come they were Ordered Ashore . . . and Taught How
to Use the firelock by Major Gilman. . . ."

Despite such command problems, and the fact that
the fleet was delayed because of ice in Gabarus Bay, the
attacking force finally appeared before Louisbourg on the
thirtieth of April, and the siege began. It lasted nearly
seven weeks, and during that time the amateur militarists
from New England performed some outstanding feats.

There were genuine hardships that were by no means solely due to the terrain, or even to French resistance either by land or sea. According to one anonymous diarist of the campaign, on May 20, "The variety of Fatigues and the unwholesomeness of the Climate with the poor accomodation—etc. were too hard for the men at last who were taken down in great Numbers with Fever and Fluxes—so that at some times near 1,500 were uncapable of Duty."

As a matter of fact, according to the commander himself, about this time only 2,100 out of 4,000 men were fit for duty. Fever and the bloody fluxes were responsible for the morbidity in his command. This was hardly inexplicable considering the housing, which was execrable, and the food, which was mostly moldy pork and bread, and now and then similarly spoiled beans and peas. The methods of food preservation employed must have made every day a feast day for *Salmonella* and typhoid organisms.

It is well established among historians that the French surrendered Louisbourg because of lack of ammunition and because of a certain lack of enthusiasm for their cause. Perhaps this totally accounts for the capitulation, but at least one observer intimates that the defenders, too, had their problems with disease. And so he states, ". . . while I was in the Citty I went to See the Place where they Buried their Dead . . . Since we Besieg'd—There was Such Numbers Kill'd and that Died—with Sickness, that they Digg'd A Hole about twelve feet Square (and about as Deep) Where they threw in all together, and without Coffins I was told. . . ." The various accounts agree that there were relatively few deaths from gunfire in the fortress. Apparently the fevers and fluxes were prevalent in "the Citty" as well as among the attacking host.

In any event Louisbourg was in the hands of the amateur soldiery from Massachusetts, the troops and inhabitants of the fortress were all embarked for France and the town was now in full possession of the victors.

Over two centuries later, the Colonial Dames may look on this event as a glorious achievement, but to the con-

querors of Louisbourg, it was a dreary triumph. The town
was a shambles and there was little shelter available. It
rained interminably. The weather was cold. Tents were
flimsy and practically useless. Huts built of turf soon dis-
solved into masses of mud. As so often happens during a
siege, the town had become so filthy that the wells were
contaminated and the drinking water was literally a
poison. As one well-known Boston physician described the
situation ". . . the people died like rotten sheep." And so
they did. For days and weeks from fifteen to twenty or
more every day were carried out the Maurepas Gate to the
cemetery behind the town, until as Shirley noted the next
spring, 890 men had died during that terrible winter.

The original plan had been for relief regiments from
Gibraltar to garrison the fort during the winter, but the
coast appeared forbidding to those warriors, and they had
spent the chilly season in Virginia. If the French could
have attacked during this period of travail, Louisbourg
would have again been in their hands. But as it was, the
New Englanders held out until relief did come, and then
went home, having won the first major military success in
the long struggle with the French for North America.

It was not the intent that the capture of Louisbourg
should end the campaign against Canada. In addition to
the three British regiments that finally relieved the colonials in April after their ghastly winter, London had promised five battalions more under Lt. General St. Clair,
together with a fleet to aid in the operations. The British
force and levies from New England would sail up the St.
Lawrence, and another contingent, with Shirley at the
head, would set out for Montreal by the familiar Lake
Champlain route. This time there was great enthusiasm
due to the success of the Massachusetts expedition of the
previous year, and the provincial assemblies of seven colonies voted an amazing total force of forty-three hundred
men.

Again the situation was fouled up. The Duke of New-
castle, who was calling the shots in Britain, also had a

European war on his hands. General St. Clair was sent instead to the coast of Brittany, where he failed to capture a post that offered to surrender. After this astounding paradox in military manipulation, perhaps it is just as well that the North American scene was not further clouded with operatives of such competence. However, Shirley decided that even if an all-out campaign was not in the cards, at least he could take Crown Point. This campaign was abandoned when it suddenly became apparent that the enemy also had plans, and had power.

In the field of modern public health, there is an aphorism to the effect that the real victories are the epidemics that never occur. If as historians we were to reverse this truism, we might opine that in the realm of military sanitation, the great disasters were oftentimes the battles that were never engaged. An outstanding, an almost forgotten such incident was about to take place.

At this time the armies of France under Saxe, the greatest general of the age, were triumphant in Europe; and her navy, in a coalition with that of Spain, was a formidable fighting force. That her great pride in North America, the mighty fortress of Louisbourg, should be snatched from her possession by a mere mob of provincials, without even professional leadership, was more than the honor of France could abide. Despite the burdens of a concurrent continental struggle, it was determined in Paris that Louisbourg should be retaken and the detested New England coast laid waste in retribution.

In the spring of 1746 the news reached Boston that the town was in grave danger, and suddenly its inhabitants began to realize that war was a two-way street and that the capture of Louisbourg was not merely a glorious adventure, but an irritating and humiliating wounding of the national pride of a world power, and retaliation might be grievous. The people were terrified. War was something to be waged on others' doorsteps, not at home. Troops that were on the march to Crown Point on Lake Champlain were immediately called home. The militia from the farms and villages for forty miles around to the number of eight thousand soon swarmed into Boston, and Connecticut agreed to furnish several thousand more. The defenses of Castle William were beefed up, cannons were hauled out and emplanted on the islands in the mouth of the harbor. The channel was obstructed with sunken hulks and a boom.

There was ample reason for the alarm. The French were angry and were in earnest. Fitting out in Brest and Rochford was a formidable fleet of ships-of-the-line, frigates, fireships, and transports that composed nearly half of the entire navy of France. In command was the Duc d'Anville, of the ancient house of La Rochefoucauld, and with 6,000 sailors and 3,500 soldiers, he sailed from the Isle d'Aix on June 20, 1746, with the mightiest collection of armament yet to set forth for the New World.

Seldom have the misfortunes of war so little depended on warfare. Headwinds and storms brought damage and delay at the start. Some of the ships were slow, so that the whole fleet must linger to keep pace with the laggards. Near the Azores a dead calm persisted for days. Another interruption was a fierce thunderstorm, during which several ships were struck. On one of these unfortunate vessels the lightning exploded a cargo of munitions, and more damage and casualties resulted. Then, to cap it all, "A febrile contagion" put in an appearance. We can only guess what it was, but the circumstances, the timing, and the high mortality make typhus the likeliest suspect. The interminable voyage dragged on and on. Some of the ships held more sickly than fit. Fifty bodies a day, for days on end, were hauled from the dismal holds and tossed into the Atlantic. Many of the ships ran short of food, so that even the sick had only a few biscuits each day.

At last, on the 14th of September the disconsolate fleet sighted Sable Island, off the coast of Nova Scotia. This proved to be scant relief. Their miseries had scarcely begun. Fogs and unfamiliar shoals plagued the captains, and then a terrific storm battered the fleet once more. One

transport went down with all aboard, others were dis-
masted and all were scattered. Finally the weather cleared,
and the Admiral's flagship captured a small English vessel
with a pilot on board. This individual was persuaded to
guide the French fleet into the harbor of what is now
Halifax, then known as Chibucto. It is true the pilot was
offered an alternative sporting proposition, namely to let
him find out how far he could swim with a cannon ball tied
to each foot.

The original grand strategy had called for a rendezvous at Chibucto with a smaller French fleet serving in the
West Indies, and a land force from Canada consisting of
1,700 men composed of regular troops, militia, coureurs du
bois, and Indians. Both the fleet and the army grew tired of
waiting, so the former took off for France, and the latter
returned to Quebec.

When the remains of the great French naval force
finally assembled in Chibucto Bay, a desolate wilderness
was all that greeted them. The shores were deserted, because the Micmac Indians, who had heard rumors, had no
desire to acquire the white man's epidemic. There was
nothing but the awful silence of the forest-covered hills
above the harbor to comfort the sick as the pestilence
ridden ships disembarked their feverish cargo. Scarcely
had d'Anville anchored than he himself died, "but in Such
Condition and so much Swell'd it was Generally thought
he Poysened himself. . . ." In view of his character this
seems unlikely, and if the description of his clinical condition is accurate, perhaps he was in congestive heart failure. Certainly he had been subjected to sufficient stress to
account for considerable cardiovascular deterioration. If,
perchance, such was the case, William Withering, whose
experiments proved the usefulness of foxglove as a
medication, was a mere five years old at the time, so no
French medical officer would have been able to supply his
commander with the sovereign remedy, made from the
leaf of a foxglove.

D'Anville's immediate successor took a quick, hard

look at the prospects and promptly fell on his sword. The command then devolved on Rear Admiral LaJonquiere. By this time it was apparent that the continuing ravages of disease in the fleet made an attack on Louisbourg out of the question. During the few autumn weeks spent in the harbor, there were 1,130 new graves. LaJonquiere was anxious at least to destroy Annapolis, but at the moment he had scarcely a thousand men in fighting condition, and now received the intelligence that his objective had been reinforced. Nothing but an ignominious withdrawal was possible. Five ships were loaded with the sick for the voyage back to France, but part of their cargo of misery was jettisoned every day. The remainder of the fleet was in little better shape, for the dreadful infection continued to spread so that there was danger that some transports might have their crews so decimated as to be utterly disabled in mid-ocean. The final calamity occurred when one of the homeward bound ships, the *Boree,* went aground at the very entrance of Port St. Louis, and a hundred and sixty invalids drowned within actual sight of their homeland.

Naturally the relief and joy in Boston and all along the New England coast knew no bounds. The ultimate in irony occurred, however, when the principals in Europe signed the treaty of Aix-la-Chapelle in the spring of 1748. Since neither side had been doing very well, overall, it was decided that each nation should restore its conquests. The one consequential British capture was that of Louisbourg, actually achieved by the Massachusetts colonists, while the French had taken Madras in India. These were exchanged by the articles of agreement. There are no statistics available as to the number of wigs torn off and stamped on in the streets of Boston when the terms of the treaty became known. Presumably the incidence was high.

THE FRENCH AND INDIAN WAR

By the time of the outbreak of the next phase of the long conflict, namely the French and Indian War, the pressures that had built up were somewhat changed. The English colonies shut in between the Alleghenies and the Atlantic were beginning to chafe. Other than the hard climb over the mountains or the tortuous trek through the passes, there was no road available to them to the interior. Despite these hardships, English traders, tough and truculent, were penetrating the vast area west of the rugged Appalachian range and interfering with French commerce among the Indians. Although this appeared to amount to a mere trickle, it was ominous in its implications. Over 1,100,000 whites scattered from Georgia to Maine were being denied access to the rich inland by less than 60,000 French and their savage allies. It was an explosive situation.

French domination of the waterways was absolute. They controlled the St. Lawrence, the Great Lakes, and the mouth of the Mississippi. Furthermore, they were in a strong position to repel attack, which could scarcely be made on their center unawares. There were three approaches to Montreal and Quebec. Louisbourg, again in French hands, barred the eastern access, the Lachine rapids in the St. Lawrence, the western, while Fort Frederic insolently guarded the narrows of Lake Champlain. One important and vulnerable area was the valley of the Ohio River, roughly halfway between Canada and Louisiana. English mastery of this area would cut French North America in two, whereas if the French should establish themselves firmly there, the colonists would be irrevocably hemmed in between the mountains and the sea.

In the years just prior to the outbreak of the war, many of the French interior posts suffered greatly from malaria. Then in 1751 smallpox had broken out at Detroit. "It is to be wished," says Longueuil, "that it would spread among our rebels; it would be fully as good as an army. . . . We are menaced with a general outbreak and even Toronto is in danger." But there was to be more trouble. In 1753 the French set out in earnest to fortify the sources of the Ohio, descend the river, and convert any wavering tribes to their ideology. But "fevers, lung diseases and scurvy made such deadly havoc among troops and Canadians" that the plan was thwarted. Garrisons were left and the remainder sent back to Montreal. Duquesne, the Governor of Canada, was shocked when the survivors of the expedition straggled in. "I reviewed them, and could not help being touched by the pitiable state to which fatigues and exposures had reduced them. Past all doubt, if these emaciated figures had gone down the Ohio as intended, the river would have been strewn with corpses. . . ."

When hostilities began—and incidentally, although we think the formal declaration of war is a very modern idea, war was not declared for another year—the English planned a four-pronged attack for 1755. Braddock was to move against Fort Duquesne, established a year earlier in the crucial location where the Monongahela and the Allegheny join to form the Ohio River. The other points of attack were Niagara, Crown Point (Fort Frederic), and Beausejour in Acadia.

All of this coincided with perilous days for the French. The virulent virus that had been smouldering in the north country for the past four years broke out with such fury and over such a wide area, from Quebec to Montreal and as far west as Niagara, that for a long time 1755 would be referred to in Canada as the year of the great smallpox epidemic.

The luckless General Braddock had two strikes on him before he actually set forth toward Fort Duquesne. His original difficulties were first, supply, and second, geography. Food and forage were hard to come by, wagons suddenly became scarce and expensive, and as for horses, the local farmers dragged into camp and sold to the British a collection of nags that could never have been processed into a good grade of glue.

Despite these harassments the outfit finally got started late in April, 1755. Within a short time the third problem appeared, which was bacterial. Captain Robert Cholmley's batman entered the following in his journal for "Satterday

May the 17th. This day a Capt belonging to Sir Peter
Halket's Regt dyed of a vilant Feaver which the Cuntry is
very Subject to." Illness was not confined to combatants
however, because he notes, "Sunday May the 25 . . . This
day we had no prayers, the Minister Being Sick."

On June 7 George Washington, serving as aide to
General Braddock, was writing to William Fairfax from the
camp at Will's Creek, "Tomorrow, Sir Peter Halket, with
the first brigade, is to begin his march, and on Monday the
General, with the second, is to follow. One hospital is filled
with sick, and the numbers increase daily, with the bloody
flux, which has not yet proved mortal to many." It did not
need to prove mortal to many in an army on the march to
be of the utmost military importance. A major objective of
the British forces was to arrive at Fort Duquesne before
French reinforcements, coming down from Canada, could
get there. It can scarcely be argued that an army beset
with diarrhea is capable of making speed when it is necessary to fell trees, move rocks, build a semblance of a road
with no power other than mammalian muscle, and then
haul supplies and munitions in sufficient quantity to go
into combat at the end of an arduous journey.

Within a week the Virginian himself was laid by the
heels, and he describes his situation with some feeling.
This account of his own illness, an experience obviously
shared with many others, indicates the extent to which an
affliction of this sort, so frequently treated as a joke, can
disable a military enterprise. On June 28th he wrote:

> Immediately upon our leaving the camp at George's Creek, on the
> 14th instant, from whence I wrote to you, I was seized with a
> violent fever and pain of the head, which continued without
> intermission until the 23rd, when I was relieved, by the General's
> absolutely ordering the physician to give me Dr. James's powders,
> one of the most excellent medicines in the world. It gave me
> immediate ease, and removed my fever and other complaints in
> four days time. My illness was too violent to suffer me to ride,
> therefore I was indebted to a covered wagon for some part of my
> transportation; but even in this, I could not continue far.

Dr. Robert James was a learned physician and lexicographer of London, and a friend of Samuel Johnson. His secret remedy which he had patented—a not unusual procedure for physicians of that day—presumably contained oxide of antimony and calcium phosphate, the latter derived from shavings of stag-horn. Most modern physicians, if their reputations depended on exhibiting a sovereign remedy to the general's aide in the field, would prefer, if Dr. James's powder were the only one available, to withhold the medication until the ninth day of a self-limited disease.

Braddock was beset by many logistic problems. Some of them he should have foreseen, some of them he was advised about but chose to ignore. No one, however, could have warned him in advance that his expedition would be slowed down by fever and dysentery among his troops to a bare three miles a day.

Well, almost no one. There was a man who might have predicted it. Three years before the present campaign this man had published in London, *Observations on the Diseases of the Army*. He was Sir John Pringle, Physician-General to His Majesty's Forces, and he knew whereof he spoke.

In regard to the very problem hampering Braddock at the moment, Pringle has this to say:

> In order, therefore, to preserve a purity of air in the dysenteric season, let there be some slight penalty, but strictly inflicted, upon every man that shall ease himself anywhere about the camp, but on the privies. Farther, from the middle of *July*, or from the appearance of a spreading flux, let the privies be made deeper than usual, and once a day a thick layer of earth thrown into them, till the pits are nearly full; and then they are to be well covered, and supplied by others.

Helpful as this advice might have been, it is unlikely that there was a single copy of Pringle's book anywhere in North America at the time. No American edition would appear for more than half a century to come. But the same admonition was still available in every hamlet in the colonies, and was more stringently expressed and spoken with more authority. In the twenty-third chapter of Deuteronomy, Moses lays it on the line, "You shall have a place outside the camp and you shall go out to it; and you shall have a stick with your weapons; and when you sit down outside, you shall dig a hole with it, and turn back and cover up your excrement. Because the Lord your God walks in the midst of your camp, to save you and to give up your enemies before you. . . ."

The defeat of Braddock was only one of the disappointments suffered by British arms in North America that year. Johnson, with a force of provincial troops, was to capture Crown Point, the fortress on Lake Champlain that so long had been a major threat to the northern colonies. There was a battle near Lake George in which Baron Dieskau, leader of the French, was killed, but then Johnson decided not to attack the garrison at Crown Point. Monckton was more successful. He had taken the French forts at Beausejour in June, whereupon those on the St. John River were abandoned.

The final effort of the summer was to have been the capture of Niagara. The intent was to mount the attack from Oswego, on the southern shore of Lake Ontario, but again there were problems. The commander, Shirley, had a smaller force than he had been promised, and the morale of the men rapidly deteriorated on receiving the news about Braddock. Their provisions did not arrive, and many of them, including Shirley's own son, died of a "Flux and Fever" due largely to the incredible filthiness of the camp. There were other, strictly tactical issues. Niagara lay to the westward at a distance of four or five days by boat or canoe along the south shore of the lake. Fifty miles or so across the lake to the north lay Fort Frontenac, the present site of the city of Kingston, Ontario. At Frontenac there was a potent force of French regulars and Canadians, who could fall on Oswego as soon as Shirley took off to attack Niagara. There could be **no** secret about the plans of the

English, for in Braddock's captured baggage were all the
current English military plans.

There was, therefore, nothing to do except wait until
spring to mount the attack. It was a tough winter. Food ran
low, scurvy appeared, and aid ultimately arrived one day
before the commander had determined to abandon the
fort. More than half the garrison had died of hunger or
disease, and the men were so weak that the sentries often
fell down at their posts. The supplies and reinforcements,
however, were of little avail, and the following summer
Oswego surrendered to the French.

Except for the loss of Oswego, little of any consequence happened in 1756. The British were hardly in a
position to take the offensive, because of command, supply, and personnel problems. In November, 1756, in a letter
from M. de Vaudreuil of Montreal to M de Moras, he says,
"Finally that small pox was prevailing in both the forts and
at Orange [Albany]," and in despatches from Canada in the
same year, we find the following brief but pungent refer-
ence, "This disease has committed ravages also among the
Canadians and prevented M. de Vaudreuil executing the
movements and invasions he had projected during the
winter." The Indians, too, were in bad case, for according
to Hutchinson, "In all former wars between England and
France, the Indians, upon the eastern frontiers, had taken
part with the French. The poor creatures had lately been
visited with the small pox, which is remarkably fatal to
them, and they were reduced to so small a number that the
French neglected them. . . ."

In the spring of 1757 things were looking up for the
French. The Indians had been heartened by the capture of
Oswego and by renewed activity in Canada. Montcalm,
who had arrived in North America the previous year, was
determined to attack the English on Lake George, where
they were uncomfortably close to the strategic positions of
Lake Champlain, and then perhaps take Fort Edward and
strike terror in the settlement of Albany.

Fort William Henry on Lake George had long had a

reputation as a sickly post. It was situated between the lake and a swamp, and its sanitation would not support the name. The English were well aware that this fort would be a prime objective and the installation had been reinforced, but Montcalm was in earnest. The siege lasted for several days. Inside the fort there were more than three hundred killed and wounded, but the principal source of casualties was smallpox. The casemates were crowded with the sick and the dying. It was nothing less than a raging epidemic, and the situation was such that there was no recourse other than surrender. After the capitulation many of the captives were massacred, but the Indians, ravenous for scalps, could not contain themselves. In the graveyard of the fort were hundreds of fresh corpses, promptly ex-humed by the savages for their epicranial trophies. But many of their post-mortem victims were not casualties of battle but rather of variola. The virus will survive under these conditions, and it will strike down anyone who is not immune. Again there was a violent exacerbation of the epidemic among the Indians. Again they were diseased and demoralized. Again their assistance to the French was largely lost.

A far greater disaster, from the medical military point of view, was to strike in Canada. On several occasions during the previous two years, transports had arrived at Quebec from the homeland bringing soldiers, many of whom were sick, and who conveyed their infections to the civilian population, but these were merely preludes to the crescendo that was about to be reached. In the spring of 1757 a fleet under the command of M. Dubois de la Mothe sailed from Rochefort for Louisbourg. There was sickness on board, and so the ships touched at Brest and four hundred were sent ashore, too ill for active service. On May third the fleet put out to sea, arriving at Louisbourg on June 28th. In a short time the sickness, almost certainly typhus, appeared in all the fleet and had spread in the fortress. Nor was the infection to be confined to Louis-bourg. From Quebec on the 25th of October, M. Doreil wrote to M. de Paulmy, "All the scourges are at one and the same time afflicting this poor country; which is on the verge of being itself destroyed, if measures as prompt as they are just be not adopted for its relief. Upon the troubles of war has supervened an epidemic disease which has been introduced by the ships that brought the soldiers. It has already committed great ravages and apprehensions are entertained for the consequences." About this same time Montcalm was reporting that there were 2,600 in Quebec hospitals, about a fifth of whom died.

In 1758 the turn of fortune became apparent. Smallpox and typhus among the French had bought time for the British in North America, and time was all they would need. William Pitt had come to power and the organizing genius of Pitt would soon make itself felt far away across the Atlantic. General Amherst took Louisbourg and its sick, numbering between a thousand and twelve hundred, in July. The following month Bradstreet captured the feebly garrisoned Fort Frontenac, and in November General Forbes, although practically an invalid from an abdominal ailment that would cause his death, arrived at Fort Duquesne and found it abandoned by the French.

As the new year began, Montcalm and his forces were in a desperate plight. The capture of Louisbourg had disrupted communications with Paris, the harvest of the previous season had been poor, much of the cattle and some of the horses had been killed for food, and again there was sickness in the embattled city. Within a few months the General Hospital was overflowing with sick and wounded, and all the sheds, barns, and garrets were filled with misery.

General James Wolfe, who had been on Amherst's staff at the capture of Louisbourg the previous year, arrived back there from London and in May had assembled the armament he was to command for the reduction of Quebec. Wolfe was a tall, ungainly redhead, thirty-two years old and already a victim of arthritis and kidney stones. Any medical officer in any modern army would throw up his hands and refuse to certify such a decrepit specimen for promotion. In view of the outcome, it is fortunate for the empire that physical examinations were not in vogue in the British army in 1759.

By the end of June Wolfe had established his forces on the Isle d'Orleans and commenced the siege of Quebec. Before long the commander was ill. According to Parkman, "He lay in his quarters, helpless in bed, his singular and most unmilitary features haggard with disease and drawn with pain, no man could have looked less the hero. . . ." But he recovered sufficiently to lead the midnight landing at what is still known as Wolfe's cove and up the cliff to the Plains of Abraham where both he and his adversary would receive their fatal wounds that same day. And so it was on the land that is now a peaceful park, covered with flowers and shrubs, close by the busy city of Quebec, a few thousand men on each side with muskets and bayonets determined the destinies of vast areas of land and its inhabitants, and of millions of people yet to be born.

In one sense the affair had not been settled. After the fall of the city the natural question was should the conquerors keep it or destroy it? The decision was to hold on and defend the prize against any attacks that might be made by Levis, the French commander still in the field. The British command devolved on General Murray. It was another long, hard, cold Canadian winter. The attrition among the troops was severe, with the effective strength of the garrison reduced to less than half those present. There were no fresh provisions; scurvy, fever, and dysentery wreaked havoc among the troops. Of roughly 7,000 men who had been left at Quebec in the previous autumn, hardly more than 3,000 were fit for duty by the end of April, 1760. About 700 had been buried for the winter, at least, in the huge snowdrifts. There was no human strength to dig graves in the wintry earth, frozen to the consistency of granite.

The French were well aware, through their multitude of spies, that Murray's sick list was as long as his roster of

fit-for-duty. An attack was made, but the French themselves lacked the needed power and Murray held them off,
and his "half-starved, scorbutic skeletons" were still in
possession of Quebec when relief ultimately arrived in
May.

THE REVOLUTION

Many thoughtful volumes have been written detailing
the background of the origins of our revolt against Britain.
It would scarcely be in good taste to oversimplify the issues
in a few sentences in a work of this sort. As soon as the
French and Indian War was over, however, the outcome
that was about to develop was foreseen by the cynical but
highly civilized French leaders. The English colonists in
North America had relatively little in common with one another. The social strata or the nationalities from which they
sprung, the climate they endured, their culture and their
mode of making a living were all quite different in Boston,
in Pennsylvania, and in Virginia. Now that they no longer
had cause to fear French assaults on their commerce, the
traditional ties with the mother country, which suddenly
began to carry a burdensome price in the form of Sugar
Acts and Townshend duties, began to appear unnecessary.
The thought even occurred to some of the patriots that
they were being taxed without being represented in the
levying assembly. In any case, scarcely more than seven
years elapsed between the signing of the Peace of Paris
and the Boston Massacre. Forces were already in motion
which would culminate in another five years in open military revolt. The colonies and the mother country were on
collision course.

Soon after Bunker Hill the decision was made by Congress to attack Canada. This was not merely because it had
become a habit over nearly a century to launch attacks
against the northern colonies when there was nothing
better to do. There were genuine political and military
reasons for the move. For one thing, the Quebec Act,

passed by Parliament in 1774, contained among its provisions the extension of the boundaries of the province to include all the land north of the Ohio River between the Allegheny Mountains and the Mississippi. This particularly infuriated Massachusetts, Connecticut, and Virginia, which had viewed this territory as largely their own. From the strategic angle, if the British could be driven out of Boston, they would then have no foothold on the Atlantic coast nearer than Halifax as a base of operations. This would be especially harrowing for an attacking army requiring reinforcement and supply by sea from a great distance. There were other considerations. With the St. Lawrence in American hands and the two principal cities of Quebec and Montreal occupied by the revolutionaries, New England would be in no danger of attack from the north; and furthermore the historic and highly vulnerable highway of the Richelieu River and Lake Champlain would be slammed shut, so that the royalist invaders could not split New England from the remaining rebellious colonies.

To achieve the desired conquest there would once again be a pincers approach, but this time with an important and necessary variation. There was no colonial navy available for a repetition of the many previous grand fleet attacks up the St. Lawrence. Furthermore, the British were in command of the sea. This time the right arm of the pincers was to be formed by a little army that would assemble in Cambridge, march to Newburyport, embark there and go up the coast to the mouth of the Kennebec. Then they would travel another forty-odd miles upriver to about the present site of Augusta, and then in small boats and on foot, up the Kennebec and the Dead River, across the Height of Land and down the Chaudiere to Quebec. The left arm of the pincers was the conventional approach, from Ticonderoga northward on Lake Champlain to the Richelieu River to the St. Lawrence and Montreal. This campaign was under the command of Major General Philip Schuyler, with Brigadier General Richard Montgomery second-in-command. At the outset, Schuyler was ill "with a bilious fever and violent rheumatick pains" and got no farther than Isle au Noix in the Richelieu River. At this point his illness worsened, and he returned to Ticonderoga. Montgomery took charge of a mixed collection of terror-stricken troops who had much disease and little discipline. Despite great obstacles, he obtained the surrender of the fort at St. Johns and captured Montreal.

There is no point in retelling here the story of the expedition to Quebec. No more succinct or vivid a description of such an episode occurs anywhere in the language than that of the commander himself, Benedict Arnold, written from Point aux Trembles November 27, 1775.

> Thus in about eight weeks we completed a march of near six hundred miles, not to be paralleled in history; the men having with the greatest fortitude and perseverance hauled their batteaux up rapid streams, being obliged to wade almost the whole way, near 180 miles, carried them on their shoulders near forty miles, over hills, swamps and bogs almost impenetrable, and to their knees in mire; being often obliged to cross three or four times with their baggage. Short of provisions, part of the detachment disheartened and gone back; famine staring us in the face; an enemy's country and uncertainty ahead. Notwithstanding all these obstacles, the officers and men inspired and fired with the love of liberty and their country, pushed on with a fortitude superior to every obstacle and most of them had not one day's provision for a week.

The wearisome march was one thing—military conquest would be quite another.

Modern expeditionary forces are usually accompanied and encumbered by a motley collection of reporters and commentators, whose sufferings are modestly mentioned in their dispatches and generously indemnified by their royalties. Such activities were not customary in Arnold's time, but he does seem to have enlisted an unusually large proportion of diarists and journalists. One of these, Caleb Haskell of Newburyport, made a portentous entry in his diary shortly after arriving within sight of the objective.

December 6th, Wednesday. The most of the army has arrived. We are getting in readiness to lay siege to Quebec. The small pox is all around us, and there is great danger of its spreading in the army. There are Spies sent out of Quebec every day, and some taken every day, both men and women.

The account continues:

December 16th, Saturday. Had but little firing today. We had one man killed with grape shot. I am unwell, and have been for three days unfit for duty.

December 17th, Sunday. I was ordered to the hospital. A bad storm: could not go.

December 18th, Monday. Myself and four more of our company were carried to the Nunnery hospital. All still on both sides.

December 19th, Tuesday. Today three of those who came to the hospital with me broke out with the small pox; I have the same symptoms.

December 20th, Wednesday. This morning my bedfellow, with myself, were broke out with small pox; we were carried three miles out in the country out of the camp; I am very ill.

December 21st, Thursday. The small pox spreads fast in our army.

Haskell and many of his comrades had not recovered in time to join the assault, the following week, in which the combined but enfeebled forces of Montgomery and Arnold tried to take the city by storm. The attackers were driven off, Montgomery was killed and Arnold wounded in the leg.

Following this setback a semblance of a siege was maintained, and a handful of reinforcements appeared, so that by the middle of March, Arnold could count 617 rank and file in addition to some not too trustworthy Canadians under Colonel James Livingston. But in the meantime smallpox had put at least four hundred of Arnold's men in hospital, and food, supplies and munitions were lacking both in Montreal and in the siege forces before Quebec.

On the second day of April, General David Wooster arrived with additional men that increased the American force to two thousand. The wounded Arnold went to Mon-

treal and Wooster took command at Quebec. The next
month Wooster was superseded by General John Thomas,
who faced a difficult situation when he looked over his
command. His army had been built up, by this time, to
2,500, but because of discharges, desertions and deaths,
he was down to a roster of 1,900, of whom no more than
1,000, including officers, were fit for duty. Of these, the
enlistment time of 300 had already expired, and another
200 were undergoing inoculation to immunize them
against smallpox, which meant that for some weeks they
were unavailable for action. He had no more than 500
troops that could be relied on. The facts of the matter were
that a mere ghost of an army was attempting to lay siege
against a stronghold.

Early in May the British were reinforced. General John
Burgoyne arrived with a strong force of Irish and English
regiments as well as two thousand German mercenaries.
This was overpowering to the feeble besiegers, and after a
sally from the fortress the Americans fled, leaving at the
mercy of the victors some two hundred who were too sick
to flee.

The retreat from Canada comprises one of the grim-
mest episodes in the annals of American military history. A
defeated army is a heart-rending sight under any circumstances, but this was a defeated army on foot or in small
boats, traveling through a hostile country, harassed by a
victorious enemy at its rear, and hampered by desperately
ill men who had left their sodden beds of straw rather than
remain as prisoners. There were not enough boats for the
effective men and supplies, urgently needed should a rear-
guard action be required. Forty miles up the St. Lawrence
at Deschambault, General Thomas temporarily halted the
rout, but after a council of war it was determined to withdraw the fragments of the army to Sorel at the mouth of
the Richelieu.

On June second, while his men were on the march to
Chambly, General Thomas himself died of the smallpox.
General John Sullivan, sent from New York to take over

the command, discovered he was in an impossible plight. "I found myself at the head of a dispirited Army, filled with horror at the thought of seeing their enemy . . . Small pox, famine and disorder had rendered them almost life-less . . . I found a great panick . . . among both officers and soldiers . . . no less than 40 officers begged leave to resign . . . However I might fortify Sorel, my men would in general leave me."

In the meantime Arnold in Montreal appreciated the indisputable fact that he was in a trap and so withdrew with his small contingent from the city and joined Sullivan's fleeing mob on the Richelieu, where Schuyler had sent them some boats. So the frightened, famished, feverish men crammed themselves aboard and pushed off for Isle aux Noix just in time to escape the advance patrols of the British.

Isle aux Noix in the Richelieu River was a revolting bit of terrain covered by brush and swamps and swarming with mosquitoes and black flies. There was little shelter, little food, and no medicine. Of the several thousand fugitives who landed on the island, at least one-quarter had smallpox, and before long most of the others had dysentery or malaria. Death was everywhere and huge common graves were filled every day. Finally the remainder was re-embarked, and those with strength to pull an oar brought the helpless and moribund back to Crown Point early in July.

Once more the virus of smallpox had come to the defense of Canada.

THE WAR OF 1812

The War of 1812 is one that almost everyone would prefer to forget. That includes, surprisingly, both those who presumably won it as well as those who presumably lost it. It is still difficult, after more than a century and a half, to be certain why it was fought. Undoubtedly there were harassments created by a great maritime power in

the process of expanding an empire, and yet the Administration in Washington had serious doubts as to whether
the enemy should be Britain or France. Certainly there
were the war hawks in Congress, of whom the leader,
Henry Clay, would shout, "The conquest of Canada is in
your power. . . Is it nothing to acquire the entire fur-trade
connected with that country . . . ?" And yet the same
Congress that heard such oratory with delight voted down
the proposal of the naval committee to appropriate seven
and a half million dollars to build a new navy and turned a
deaf ear to Gallatin's urgent appeal for new taxes.

What no nation can afford to forget are the moments
in its history it would prefer not to remember. Shame and
defeat are just as valuable elements in a nation's annals as
are victory and conquest. It is from errors that lessons are
learned as well as from triumphs.

In any case, there would be no point in going into
detail regarding the various campaigns on the northern
border and on the lakes if it were not that once again the
element of disease played a significant role in the defense
of Canada.

In this conflict it was of no particular advantage to the
country that at the outbreak of hostilities the secretary of
war was a physician. Dr. William Eustis had served as a
surgeon during the Revolution. He had been appointed
secretary of war in 1809, and one of his supporters in
Congress had proffered the encomium that he was at least
as good as the secretary of the navy. Under the circumstances there could have been no feebler kudos. He was also
described as one who "consumes his time in reading
advertisements of petty retailing merchants to find where
he may purchase one hundred shoes or two hundred
hats. . . ."

Eustis, while making his various inspection tours of
the military posts, was occasionally called in as a consul-
tant on some surgical problem confronting the hospital
staff. It must have been a shattering experience for an invalided soldier suddenly to discover himself being gravely

pummeled and pawed in the most private parts of his anatomy by the secretary of war.

A multitude of serious problems faced Madison when war was declared. For one thing, he was the first casualty. He developed an intermittent fever in June and was confined to his bed for weeks. Dolly was beside herself and even at the end of July was still watching over him as she would an infant. His worst quandary, however, was not his own health. On June 6, 1812, the war department's return of officers and men totalled 6,744. These were widely scattered over a huge area and engaged in essential garrison duty. There was a desperate shortage of officer material all the way up to, and especially at, the top. Thirty years had passed since Yorktown, the Indian fighting and the local citizens' rebellions occurring since then were poor schooling for field grade officers. The administrations of both Jefferson and Madison had been stingy with military appropriations, and the Military Academy at West Point was only ten years old and small for its age.

The senior commanding general was Henry Dearborn, sixty-one years old, also a physician and also a former secretary of war. (For seventeen of the first twenty-three years of this republic's existence, the secretary of war was a physician. If our military establishment could survive that handicap, no wonder, in its subsequent career, it has performed so well.) Dearborn's rheumatism was beginning to bother him, but the aspirin tablet was eight decades away. The second ranking general was William Hull, a mere fifty-nine, but Hull's arteries were as stiff as Dearborn's joints.

Another pressing major issue facing the President was the fact that there really was not the slightest concept of how to provide the men and material for a war. Naturally there were always the ancient, dog-eared plans to unshelve, dust off and re-study. Canada must be invaded! Aside from the covetous motivation to possess the fur trade, from the strategic point of view, this still made sense. If the British, currently involved with the uncertainties of the war in Europe, were to conduct a land campaign on the North American continent, they could only do it from the north. There were scarcely the fleet and men available, with the Napoleonic conflict at their back, to mount an attack against the cities along the Atlantic coast. The obvious staging area for an assault on the United States was Canada. On the other hand, to forestall such an approach, and take the initiative, an invasion from the American side was the sole recourse.

When the grand strategy was ultimately determined, the principal objective would be to move by way of the well-traveled route up Lake Champlain from a base at Albany and capture Montreal. Supporting movements would be directed from such border points as Sackett's Harbor on Lake Ontario, near where the St. Lawrence River emerges; from the Niagara River, a frontier thirty-six miles in length; and from Detroit, a village with a population then of about eight hundred.

The American plan was for Hull, at Detroit, to capture Fort Malden (at what is now Amherstburg in Ontario) while Dearborn was taking Montreal and incidentally gathering in the Niagara border posts. Then Hull would move east to join Dearborn. However, command problems promptly appeared. Hull was less than eager to invade Canada, and Dearborn never seemed quite sure in his own mind how far his authority extended. It is perfectly possible that Hull was suffering from a depressive psychosis. His record during the Revolution had been anything but that of a coward, but now, mentally and emotionally he came apart at the seams. "Conditions finally reached the point where there was scarcely anyone in the command who did not recognize that the only thing that could save the army would be a new leader." But the new leader was not forthcoming. Hull fumbled briefly and ineffectively with Fort Malden and then withdrew to the American side of the river. In August, 1812, the British General Isaac Brock, with a handful of troops, literally terrified Hull into surrendering Detroit.

In the east, for what was intended to be the principal theater of the war, General Dearborn began to assemble an army in upstate New York, with his headquarters in Albany and the camp situated across the Hudson at Greenbush. His problems were not all administrative. Men were arriving and leaving at frequent intervals and there was considerable sickness ". . . the diseases being chiefly dysentery and diarrhea, due to want of cleanliness, bad cooking and intemperance. . . ."

Dearborn's advance to the border, his inconsequential skirmish and immediate return, if mentioned at all by historians, are ordinarily polished off with a single hasty sentence. Probably that is as it should be, but if the circumstances were utterly inglorious, perhaps they were also slightly extenuating. One surgeon's mate during this campaign was a young man who would, some years in the future, become one of the brightest stars in the U.S. Army Medical Department. This was Dr. William Beaumont, and at this time in his career his most famous patient, Alexis St. Martin, was a nine-year-old boy whose gastric secretions were flowing exactly as nature intended them to do.

According to Dr. Beaumont:

Near the Middle of November 1812 the Army moved from Plattsburgh to the Province Line, 45 Deg. North, taking no tents, and destitute of covering, save a Blanket or two, lying out in open air after marching all day through the mud and water, and thus exposed to the inclemencies of the weather for a week, encampt in the woods. After which the army returned to Plattsburgh, and there encamp'd again in the woods without Tents or Huts the first night, which was very rainy and cold; the Second also was wet and windy. They then moved to Saranac, and encamped again in the woods, during which time the weather was various—warm and cold, sometimes raining, sometimes snowing—the men lying upon the cold, wet ground, and with only a fire before their tents, for two, three or four weeks. Whilst in this wretched and deplorable situation, the men were seized with Dysentery, Intermittents, Pleurisy, Peripneumony, Cynanche and Rheumatism, which made the very woods ring with coughing and groaning.

Peripneumonia was a severe epidemic disease of the lungs, with a high attack rate and a high mortality. Civilians were stricken as well as soldiers, and the physicians of the period apparently were unfamiliar with the entity. Dr. Joseph A. Gallup, who wrote a book about epidemics in early Vermont, describes the situation in these words:

> The autumn of 1812, and the winter of 1813, ushered in the most severe epidemic disease, that has ever afflicted the inhabitants of Vermont, the epidemic peripneumony, or disease of the lungs. . . . The disease appeared at the northward before it did in the country of Windsor, perhaps about one month. It appeared amongst the soldiers at Burlington, some weeks before it did amongst the inhabitants of that place. Very near the time it appeared at Burlington among the soldiers, it appeared also among the soldiers at Plattsburg and Sacketts Harbor, and also in the camp at Greenbush, opposite Albany. . . . The pestilential diathesis of the atmosphere, was not at its zenith until the first week in March. In this month it raged with its greatest severity. It is said, that many of the soldiers died in four to eight hours after the attack, and a few in two hours . . . The common fatal period was about the fourth or fifth day. . . ."

So now Detroit had fallen, the campaign against Montreal had been a fiasco, but in the meantime there had been action on the Niagara sector. Again there were command disputes. Stephen Van Rensselaer, who had been appointed to take charge of the militia in the western part of the state by the Governor of New York, was given little help either by Dearborn or by the war department, and was thoroughly scorned by Brigadier General Alexander Smyth who commanded the regulars stationed at Buffalo.

In mid-October, 1812, Van Rensselaer crossed into Canada; first, to avenge the disgrace of Detroit, and second, because just over the river and into the trees, there were some fine winter barracks that he thought might be easier to capture than to build. He crossed at Queenston, a village opposite Lewiston, seven miles upriver from General Brock's headquarters at Fort George. An American sortie under Captain John E. Wool captured Queenston heights, and during the fracas General Brock was killed.

Van Rensselaer realized that the American invading party would need help if the British brought up reinforcements, which they did. But try as he would, Van Rensselaer could not persuade the quavering militia to cross the river and come to the aid of their comrades. So the conquerors of Queenston heights were made prisoner, and the Americans lost a battle, a courageous detachment of officers and men, and much honor. The British, on their part, lost an irreplaceable combat general.

Brigadier General Smyth, at Buffalo, was now to have his brief, inglorious moment on the stage. Following a terrific barrage of Billingsgate, which did little to impress the enemy but much to embarrass his countrymen, he ordered an invasion of Canada. Boats were assembled, and one day late in November, some twelve hundred men with artillery were embarked and moved a few miles downstream to Black Rock, still on the American side, where they were ordered to disembark and eat lunch. Literally that was all that happened. Smyth announced that he required three thousand men in order to cross the river and attack the British. Probably he was right, supposedly there were four thousand regulars available; but measles and peripneumonia had flourished along the Niagara that autumn, and more than half of Smyth's army were either invalids or were dead. There simply were no more serviceable troops, so the invasion was called off and Smyth shuffled off to Buffalo and into limbo.

In the spring of 1813 the tactically successful but strategically disastrous raid on York occurred, which later would give the British sufficient excuse for burning Washington. Lake Ontario was now considered a more favorable theater of operations than the well-protected approaches to Montreal. Dearborn planned to follow the raid on York with an attack on Fort George that guarded from the Canadian side the mouth of the Niagara River as it enters Lake Ontario. He would thus clear the Niagara frontier of the British and then, by capturing Kingston, isolate Lake Erie in his rear.

The American army evacuated York on the first of May, 1813. Owing to incredibly foul winds, it took a full week for the crowded and dirty troop vessels to make the trivial passage across the lake. When the forces were finally disembarked on May eighth, they arrived, according to Dearborn's report, "in a very sickly and depressed state; a large proportion of the officers and men were sickly and debilitated."

Sicklier than any of his men was the commanding general, who at this juncture was seized with a fever, and a short time later with what sounds like an anginal attack— "a violent spasmodic attack on his breast, which has obliged him to relinquish business altogether." Fortunately for the home team his chief of staff, Colonel Winfield Scott, was in charge, and at the end of May the land forces, with the cooperation of Commodore Chauncey's fleet, captured Fort George.

During this spring season Benjamin Rush was writing some pungent comments to his friend John Adams about the whole situation, "Count Saxe says three things are requisite to make a general, viz., courage, genius, and *health*. Three of our generals are above *sixty*, a time of life in which the employments inseparable from a camp and military duty seldom fail of deranging the body and mind. Each of those generals has been laid up with sickness since their appointment, and two of them nearly in sight of the enemy."

Somehow or other the summer was wasted. It was a green army and it needed training, but there were hindrances. Dr. James Mann, a hospital surgeon serving with the forces on the frontier, wrote, "During the month of August, an uncommon proportion of the army were sick, or unfit for duty. More than one-third of the soldiers were on the sick reports. The officers shared with the privates in the prevailing diseases. Half of the medical staff attached to regiments, were also unable to perform their duty." Dr. Joseph Lovell, who later was to become, when the office was created, the first surgeon-general of the army, and who also was at Fort George that summer reported, "The diseases . . . were such as might have been expected; typhous and intermittent fevers, diarrhoea and dysentery. . . . The cases of intermittents were numerous, and generally of the tertian type." Mention of intermittents is frequent among medical reports of the time, when malaria was rife along the Great Lakes.

This was the sad state of affairs that General James Wilkinson, who replaced Dearborn, discovered when he arrived at Niagara on September fourth. Wilkinson, whose loyalty to his country had been questioned on several occasions, was far more adept at intrigue than at administration. Physically he was no rose either. He was ill almost from the moment of his arrival at Fort George, and by the time he had moved his troops to Sackett's Harbor, nearly a month later, "He was so much indisposed in mind and body," according to one officer, "that in any other service he would have perhaps been superseded in his command." The troops he brought with him could not be described as combat-ready either. According to Dr. Mann, "We shall, here, give a retrospective view of the general health of the army, when it embarked on board the flotilla at Niagara. A large proportion of the soldiers were convalescent, and could but illy endure the fatigues and exposures in open boats, during the passage down Lake Ontario. . . . While on their tedious passage, attended with great hazard and serious disaster, many of the convalescents relapsed into former, or were seized with new diseases. . . ." It is well known that exposure such as this will cause a recrudescence of malaria as well as other ailments that may have afflicted the force.

Nevertheless, on November 5, 1813, the ill-starred expedition numbering nearly three hundred boats, having safely entered the St. Lawrence River, began the descent along the historic waterway to conquer Montreal. The general was bedridden, and his troops were in poor health. Failure stared at them from both banks of the river. The British launched gunboats to harass the flotilla from the rear, and at every narrowing of the passage opened fire from the Canadian side. Finally, to dispel the nuisance, a force was landed, but at the battle of Chrystler's Farm, about eight hundred presumably healthy British soundly defeated more than twice as many Americans, and it has been reported, "Wilkinson and Morgan Lewis, the two major-generals, who were ill on their boats, never gave an order."

How fortunate it is for posterity that no doting descendant ever commissioned a statue of James Wilkinson! Imagine, instead of a pedestal, a small boat; instead of a fiery steed, a brass bed; instead of a sword, a bottle of medicine. After this disgraceful performance, Wilkinson ordered the entire contingent, the following day, to paddle a few miles up the Salmon River to French Mills into United States territory, and there go into winter quarters.

The campaigns of 1814, for our purpose, can be briefly detailed. Early in the year, Wilkinson, now stationed at Plattsburgh, marched some four thousand men a few miles over the border to attack a small post occupying a ruggedly constructed stone mill on the Lacolle River. The American artillery, consisting of two twelve-pound field guns, scarcely chipped the walls of the mill, whereupon Wilkinson with consummate courage marched back to Plattsburgh and was relieved of his command.

The final invasion, if it can be called such, was far more creditable to United States arms. The battles at Chippewa and Lundy's Lane demonstrated that properly trained, competently officered American soldiers could hold their own against equal or even superior British forces. These conflicts occurred almost literally within sight of the spray sent up by the Niagara cataract and had little effect on the outcome of the war. They did, however, represent the last time Canada would ever suffer an invasion. From the point of view of the United States, Dr. Mann pronounced the benediction, "The greatest evils, to which the army has been subjected since the war, are diseases and their consequent mortality."

4

General Washington's Other Ally

To most Americans, the Revolution means Concord and Bunker Hill; it means Bennington and Saratoga, Long Island, Valley Forge, and Yorktown. When it comes to our history, we are a provincial people and seldom if ever think of this struggle as the most significant phase of England's Second Global War. We are usually a little startled to discover that ours was a part of a conflict fought as well in Quebec, along the Mississippi, in New Orleans, at Martinique, at Panama, at Gibraltar, at Minorca, and at Poona, and Vellore in India. We are all well aware that France was involved, but seldom stop to consider that Britain was also fighting the Spaniards and the Dutch at the same time and was having difficulties approaching rupture with Frederick the Great and with Catherine of Russia.

The Revolution has been studied in minute detail by many historians and from many varying points of view. Strategy has been exhaustively described and tactics unceasingly scrutinized. The personal qualities, good and bad, of the leaders both civil and military, on both sides, have been dissected with operating microscopes. There have been detailed investigations of supply problems, finance, political corruption, and social kinetics. There have been critiques of the French alliance and the contributions of Lafayette, de Grasse and Rochambeau to the ultimate success of the rebellious colonies. All these fac-

110

tors fully warrant the attention they have been given; but General Washington had still another ally at Yorktown in the months and years that preceded that capitulation which neither he nor his contemporaries properly appreciated.

This ally was feminine and, as is so often the case, tended to be fickle in her favors toward friend and enemy. She also, at times, had assistants of her own, as will be mentioned. Nevertheless, she probably contributed as much on her own account to winning American independence as did the troops of Rochambeau, the inspiring leadership of Lafayette, or the warships commanded by de Grasse. She was small, her figure was beguiling, and she delighted in making the acquaintance of strangers. Her name was *Anopheles Quadrimaculatus*.

The intervention of France early in 1778, following the loss of Burgoyne's army the previous autumn, transformed the whole character of the war and broadened the area of conflict. From the English point of view, this was no longer merely an annoying revolt of some misguided colonists but had suddenly become an all-out war with a major power and a traditional enemy. As a result the cabinet in London was forced to embark on a combined military and political retreat in the North American theater.

In April, Sir Henry Clinton received orders to go to Philadelphia and take over the command of the British army from Howe, who was returning to England. He was also ordered to evacuate that city and concentrate his forces in New York. Immediately his troubles as commander-in-chief began. Because of insufficient naval tonnage he decided to move the troops, not, as instructed, by sea, but overland through New Jersey. It was an extremely hot summer—"Never known such weather, by the oldest inhabitant"—and what with the heat and the action brought by the Americans at Monmouth, it was an unhappy journey.

Lieutenant Montresor, an engineer with the British forces at Philadelphia, was suffering with "a Rupture" and hence was permitted to avoid the march and go with the fleet down the Delaware River. By June 23rd he was noting in his journal, "This river rather unhealthy for the Fleet, several having fallen sick and many thrown overboard." In another week they were at Sandy Hook, but the situation appears to have worsened. On July 25th appears this entry, "Return of the Sick in the General Hospital consists of Eight hundred and Fifty Men."

By midsummer Clinton had his forces garrisoned in New York, but except for a trivial episode off Newport, terminated by a storm at sea, little or nothing of military consequence happened thereafter for a full year. It is interesting to inquire why, for so long a period, the British general was sitting on his hands.

In August the diligent diarist Lieutenant Montresor was writing in New York, "Town rather unhealthy," and a few days later, "The Hospitals rather encrease wich is not very uncommon at this season. The general calculation made of the sick in our Military Hospitals is that seven men die out of every hundred." The interpretation of this statement gives rise to some difficulties, but in spite of the way it is worded, it seems to have been the custom then to relate the number of deaths to the number in the command, rather than to the number of sick. Even so, if seven out of a hundred of all personnel died, then a huge proportion of them must have been on the sick list. On August 27th Montresor wrote, "The troops more sickly than usual, the same of the Inhabitants, 'tis thought by the faculty to be owing to the bad flour."

Whatever "the faculty" may have thought, Clinton's troops were down with malaria. This importation from the Old World had long been endemic along the East coast, and before the end of the seventeenth century had even become established in New England reaching as far north as Maine and the area around Lake Champlain. During the latter part of the colonial era it began to recede, and as Noah Webster points out, visited Hartford for the last time in the eighteenth century in 1749. The reason for this recession is a bit obscure. It is easy to say that the development of agriculture and the drainage of swamps was the reason for the departure of the infecting mosquito. It is quite possible that some far more subtle biological reason accounts for the fact that "the intermittents" departed from Hartford in 1749 but were still prevalent in New York a full generation later.

That such disorders were still prevalent is well documented by the comment of Dr. Johann David Schoepff, who came to this country as surgeon of the Anspach-Bayreuth troops. "Most newcomers to this country have to pay tribute to the climate by some indisposition or other, especially if they land during the hot season of the year. Our troops arrived here in July. From that time until October most of our men were, one after another, in the hospitals of New York or in the regimental hospitals on Staaten-Eyland or at Harlam; there were very few who escaped without an attack of dysentery or fever."

In addition to the annual summer complaints of the New York region, Clinton was to have further medical problems. According to Major Carl Leopold Bauermeister, adjutant general of the Hessian forces stationed in New York, "On the 29th of August six men-of-war from Admiral Byron's fleet again came to anchor off Sandy Hook. They immediately disembarked almost two thousand sick on Staten Island." The nature of this illness is not easy to determine, but it had been a long and difficult passage and perhaps they were suffering from scurvy. A week later, again quoting Bauermeister, "Some twenty transports arrived from Cork. They brought eight months provisions and English, Anspach, and Hessian recruits, many of whom were sick and have been taken to the hospitals. Moreover, nineteen Hessian recruits died at sea." On September 21 he writes, "Each day increases the number of sick here."

Clinton's worries were not all related to the health of his command; he was also being harried from London. The ministry was now concerned with the total war picture of which the colonial revolt was only a fragment. Soon orders arrived distributing sizeable contingents of Sir Henry's forces to faraway places. The West Indies, the perennial locale of bloodshed among European powers for centuries, would again become a battleground. An expedition was to be launched against the island of St. Lucia, and for this purpose Major General Grant was detached, along with somewhat more than five thousand choice troops. Some of Sir Henry's soldiers, among them a German battalion clothed much more properly for service in northern Canada, also went to Pensacola, a worthless fortification which should have been abandoned. Another contingent embarked under command of Lieutenant Colonel Archibald Campbell for duty in Georgia and East Florida, and smaller detachments were sent for garrison duty in the Bahamas and in Halifax. All in all the naval transports subtracted some ten thousand troops from those under Sir Henry's orders, and his sole consolation was the promise from London that by early spring he would have 6,600 fresh reinforcements from Europe, and the return to his command of the five thousand men sent to the West Indies under General Grant.

During the winter there was some pleasant news. Lieutenant Colonel Campbell captured Savannah, and the British now had a valuable naval base for future action in the South. Within weeks, all remaining opposition in Georgia collapsed, and Tories flocked in to join His Majesty's army.

In the meantime, although forced by both medical and ministerial considerations into frustrating inactivity, the commander-in-chief was drawing up plans for the coming year, 1779. Although there were at that time many isolated determined resistance groups, and various organized rebel detachments, the principal military force in the colonies opposing the royal will was the Continental army quartered at West Point.

Clinton's strategy, as the days of the new year began to lengthen, was to destroy Washington's army by drawing him into a major battle, either by threatening the major American supply depots, or by a direct attack on West Point. The idea was perfectly sound, and with the discipline and firepower that Clinton anticipated would be his, the course of history would have veered sharply in an afternoon. But it was not the sort of an afternoon that Clinton or the British Empire was destined to enjoy. Instead, malevolent fate sat by and sneered.

On the first of May, 1779, and already late by the prospective military timetable prepared in London, a huge convoy of merchant ships, troop transports and victuallers, with an escort of five warships, sailed from England under Rear Admiral Arbuthnot, headed for New York. This armada had scarcely gotten under way when word reached the admiral that the French were attacking the Channel Islands. Although Arbuthnot was much more of a sea lawyer than he was a fighter, he seems to have felt that his presence at the scene of the dispute was required. He immediately ordered the convoy into port and went to investigate the matter. At Guernsey he learned that the situation was well in hand, and so, perhaps somewhat relieved, he returned to his original responsibility.

In the meantime, however, the Admiral had received intelligence that a sizeable French fleet was making up at Brest. This would provide a threat to Arbuthnot's convoy sufficient of magnitude that he must now await the arrival of twelve more ships of the line to strengthen his escort. As a result, there was more delay, so that several weeks elapsed before the troops and supplies finally departed for New York.

Unfortunately, the soldiers on board the Admiral's transports were in need of safeguards that His Majesty's entire navy could not conceivably provide. One pertinent reason was the quality of personnel then available for military service. The ministry, by this time, was having increasing difficulty in raising troops. The war was unpopular at home, particularly among the classes from which foot soldiers might be recruited. After all, many of the liberties for which their friends and relatives overseas were fighting and dying would be equally welcome and appreciated in England. Furthermore, the levies from the continent, inexpensively available up to now, were no longer so easy to come by. To fill the rapidly depleted ranks of the king's army, therefore, all possible sources must be tapped.

In those days a minor offense could get you tossed into jail, and as a rule the sentences were unduly long. Here, then, was an obvious source of available manpower. The nation's jails were raided, and the miserable convicts, long subjected to unspeakable filth and degradation, and understandably grateful for the opportunity to breathe fresh air and see the sun again, were stuffed into uniforms and hustled aboard the transports. The jailbirds, however, did not come alone. They brought with them the vermin that had shared their dungeons for the tedious months and years of their imprisonment.

Typhus fever, as it is now called, can be recognized from descriptions of contemporary observers as a scourge that has afflicted mankind at least since the end of the fifteenth century. Under the name of "camp fever" it has castigated armies, as "ship fever" it has devastated fleets and as "jail fever" it has slain countless prisoners. On several occasions it demonstrated its contempt for the courts of law by being responsible for the Black Assizes. A survey begun in 1773 of the dark, dank dungeons of England had shown that jail fever was a frequent cause of death among the inmates of practically every jail in the country. Considering the conditions under which they served their terms, it is not surprising that prisoners characteristically gave off a "noisome smell" when they ultimately appeared above ground; and one fond theory held by the do-gooders of the day was that a little ventilation was all that would be required to eliminate this embarrassing affliction. Many long and dreary years must pass before it would be realized why the feeble ventilators installed by the reformers had succeeded in accomplishing so little.

The organism responsible for typhus fever is transmitted to man by lice. The body louse carries the infection from one human being to another. As might well be imagined, Arbuthnot's fleet became an ideal breeding ground for the disease. There were enough jailbirds on board— whether genuine criminals or merely poor debtors made no difference—and an ample supply of lice and a sufficient cargo of the infecting organism *Rickettsia prowazeki* to start things going in a big way. A long, hot summer aboard crowded, filthy troop ships where baths and clean clothing were undreamed of, could produce only one awful result. More than one hundred men died on that terrible voyage to New York, and by the time the convoy came to anchor, nearly eight hundred more were ill. Worse yet, the contagion spread so rapidly through the garrison that within six weeks, literally thousands were on the sick list in New York. Clinton was aghast. "Reinforcements came not till the 28th August, and then with such a pestilential fever as sent 6000 men to the hospital and put me *hors de combat*."

This was by no means the end of Sir Henry's current frustrations. They were to be further compounded by his failure to gain back the large numbers of men he had sent to distant sectors the previous year, presumably on loan. Many of these men would never receive another earthly assignment.

Earlier in 1779 the commanding general at St. Lucia had written in utter desperation to London, "Without bark we should not have a man fit for duty in three months; but the hospital at New York would not give so much as I looked for." The returns in this command for 5 April show 3,300 fit for duty, 1,350 sick. There were 100 deaths between March 31 and April 24. Then, when it would have been possible to return some soldiers to Clinton, British inferiority at sea prevented the transportation of four battalions. Again the sickly season arrived and the dwindling forces at St. Lucia began to fall down fast. Returns for 19 September, 1779, showed 1,137 fit for duty, 510 sick; 29 October, 933 fit, 500 sick; 30 December, 685 fit, 576 sick.

The rapid diminution of the totals is of course due to deaths.

Pensacola was a complete disaster. Personnel were unsatisfactory, equipment was unsuitable, and military intelligence was conspicuous by its absence. The Spaniards had little trouble mopping up that situation. That left Georgia, and here the expedition was a military success but the forces there were in great difficulty as can be seen from the comments of Dr. Robert Jackson, a British regimental surgeon serving with the troops:

> [The regiment] was employed in long and almost continual marching, till the latter end of April [1779], when, encamping at Ebenezer, on the Savanna river, the intermitting fever soon made its appearance, and spread so rapidly, that before the end of June, very few remained, not only in this regiment, but even in the garrison, who had not suffered more or less from this raging disease. . . . I left the garrison of Ebenezer in the beginning of July, and went directly to Savanna, where the same epidemic prevailed. . . . From Savanna, I went to Beaufort in the beginning of August. The fever, which usually prevails at this season of the year, in all the southern provinces of North America, was then epidemic among the troops who were stationed on this island. . . . This epidemic was still acquiring force, when the outposts were summoned to the defense of Savanna. Its progress was, in some measure, suspended during the active service of the siege. The enemy, however, had no sooner retired from before the place, than a fever began to rage with violence, which carried off prodigious numbers, particularly of the foreign troops. . . .

Meanwhile the situation in the north was scarcely any better. In November Major Bauermeister was reporting to his superiors in Germany:

> If only this pernicious ague and putrid fever would let up, General Clinton could undertake a great deal with the troops. But the misery prevailing here cannot be described; it must be seen. Many officers and servants are sick in bed. . . . Of the officers in von Mirbach's Regiment only Major von Wilmowsky, Captain Rodemann, and Lieutenants Wissenmuller and von Biesenroth are well; the rest are deathly ill. Some of them have had from three to five relapses. To increase this misery, the surgeons and women have been taken with fever, too. . . .

So, in that fatal year of 1779 Clinton's last hope had faded. He would never face Washington in a decisive battle and he would never crush the spirit of American independence in a single overwhelming blow. The reasons, strangely enough, were such unforeseen and unmilitary ones as typhus on shipboard and in New York, and malaria in the southern colonies, in the West Indies and in his own command. Yet despite the vexations that assailed him and the inadequacy of his force, Clinton was continually receiving letters from Lord George Germain urging him to undertake offensives here, there, and everywhere. It is small wonder that the general in a frenzy replied on one occasion, "For God's sake, my Lord, if you wish me to do anything, leave me to myself, and let me adapt my efforts to the hourly change of circumstances."

In this fashion, nearly all the year 1779 had slipped away with little of note having been accomplished. As the autumn winds began to blow, and the enervating fevers in New York abated, it was apparent that aggressive action was now feasible and the time had come to mount an offensive.

That October a French fleet under d'Estaing had failed to regain Savannah from the British and so had abandoned the attempt and sailed away. Clinton now decided that the opportunity was at hand for the complete subjugation of the South. Since Georgia was firmly in Loyalist hands, he planned a campaign that would be initiated in South Carolina and move through North Carolina and on into Virginia. The first objective was to take Charleston, establish a base, and then move inland. He was confident, in view of the previous success farther south, that Loyalist support in the entire area would forthwith swing to his banner and the revolt in those colonies would be crushed.

Embarkation day was December 26, and with Lord Cornwallis as second-in-command, Clinton sailed south to Charleston with 8,500 rank and file. It was a rough trip on a wintry sea. Men, horses, equipment, and ships were lost, but even so the expedition arrived in condition to lay siege to the city. It was a long engagement, and Governor Rutledge of South Carolina called for the local militia to come to the defense of the city. The patriots, however, demurred. They were afraid that if they were cooped up in Charleston they might be subjected to an outbreak of smallpox. On the 12th of May the city fell to the invaders and thus began a phase of the American Revolution that may be unique in military annals. Seldom, if ever, would it be possible to discover a similar series of events in wartime whereby the defeated could see their way clear to advance and the victorious be compelled to retreat.

After Charleston was in British hands, the campaign to occupy the interior of South Carolina became a major objective. In a short time, a strongly held line of posts ran across the northern rim of the colony through Camden, a principal base, to the fort called Ninety-six, while garrisons at Georgetown, Charleston, Beaufort, and Savannah held the seacoast. By the end of May what little resistance remained in South Carolina had been completely eliminated by the energy and aggressiveness of that intrepid British cavalry officer Banastre Tarleton. The situation now appeared to be well in hand, so at this point Clinton returned to New York and left Cornwallis in command of the southern theater.

The new commander inherited some nasty problems. The work up to now had been done entirely in the winter and in the spring, but the apparent ease of the campaign so far in South Carolina was not to be taken as an indicator of the course of the rest of the conquest. Tarleton himself groused:

> the heat of the summer, the want of stores and provisions and the unsettled state of Charleston and the country impeded the immediate invasion of North Carolina. . . . The legion dragoons were directed to keep the communications open between the principal posts of this extended cantonment: This service injured them infinitely more than all the preceding moves and actions of the campaign, and though hitherto successful against their ene-

mies in the field, they were nearly destroyed in detail by the patroles and detachments required of them during the intense heat of the season.

It might be noted at this point that "the heat of the season" and "the climate" were favorite etiologic excuses used both by line officers and regimental surgeons to explain the fevers that beset the soldiery, and sometimes themselves. Heat, climate, swamps, miasma—other than these, there simply were no satisfactory explanations for the ague for a full century to come.

While all this was going on, the American Congress, much to the disgust of George Washington, had sent General Gates to the Carolinas to take command of the southern department of the colonial army. The first objective of Gates was to destroy a detachment of the enemy under the command of Lord Rawdon and take Camden. There were two serious obstacles in his way. One was the terrain, the other was Rawdon.

The first problem was that the route Gates proposed to follow ran through an area sparsely inhabited and therefore thinly supplied with provisions, but well supplied with deep swamps alternating with deep sand. Furthermore, to add to the discomfiture of military forces on the march, the land was crossed by brooks and streams, all of which might, by a few hours' heavy rain, become impassable. Even more important was the stark fact that previous enemy journeys in the neighborhood had succeeded in depleting the region of its scant stores of food and forage. Finally, the Cross Creek country, which the route would traverse, was the area in all the South most inimical to the cause of the colonial rebellion.

Gates's other problem was Rawdon, unquestionably the most able combat officer that Cornwallis had, but also probably capable enough to be a welcome subordinate to any field officer anywhere.

At this juncture, however, Rawdon was not compelled to face Gates alone. Cornwallis hastened up from Charleston to join him and together they would meet the colonists' threat. At this point the Americans prepared for battle in a fashion unique in our military annals. It is just as well. One such experience is enough in the chronicles of any nation. The night before the battle some meat and corn meal had been procured for the troops; and Gates, who had never stopped preening himself about the triumph at Saratoga for which he had been given the undeserved credit, had an idea. This in itself should have been a warning, but military organization being what it is, when the commanding general has a whim, neither logic, common sense, nor even professional knowledge is likely to prevail. Gates's happy suggestion was, instead of providing the soldiery with the customary allotment of rum, to issue instead a wonderful substitute. This would be a gill of molasses from the hospital stores for every man in the outfit. Naturally, the order was obeyed. So the night before the battle of Camden the Americans ate voraciously of half-cooked meat and half-baked bread with a dessert of corn meal mush mixed with molasses. This, as one non-com described it, "served to purge us as well as if we had taken jalap." All night long the men were on the march, and all night long they were breaking ranks precipitously to pause in the underbrush beside the road. This certainly was not by any means the sole deciding factor of the battle of Camden, but it undoubtedly contributed to one of the most disastrous defeats an American army ever suffered.

At last, with Gates's army scattered and destroyed, Cornwallis was in a position to move into North Carolina. Georgia and South Carolina at his back were firmly in Loyalist hands. Neither in front of him nor on his flanks was any consequential American military force to interfere with his conquest. What did interfere, however, was the ubiquitous mosquito.

According to Dr. Jackson, the British regimental surgeon previously quoted,

> In the beginning of June the whole of the regiment arrived at Camden in perfect health . . . (and) was sent to occupy a post at the Cheraws, on the river Pedee. In a fortnight or three weeks, the intermitting fever began to show itself. It spread so rapidly,

that before the end of July, when the post was abandoned, few
were left who had not felt its influence. . . . The approach of the
enemy made it necessary that the post should be withdrawn; but
there was much difficulty in accomplishing it. Two thirds of both
officers and men were unable to march; and it was not possible,
in the situation in which we were placed, to find waggons sufficient to carry them . . . [so it was necessary] to convey some part
of them to Georgetown by water. . . . During the month of
August, and a great part of September, the army remained encamped near Camden. The weather was excessively hot, and
fevers were frequent, sometimes malignant and dangerous. . . .
In the months of October and November relapses were
numerous. . . .

To the commander, Jackson's lament was the mere
wailing and teeth gnashing of that ever-present source of
gloom and foreboding, the medical officer. Cornwallis was
eager to be on the move, and he rationalized that a change
of locale would benefit the health of the troops. In September he broke camp. He split his force into two divisions—
one, under him, would move up the east side of the
Wateree River; the other, under Tarleton, would go up the
west bank. The scarcity of forage in the area was the main
reason for this temporary separation. This division of forces
for reasons of supply was to have most awkward repercus-
sions. The two divisions were supposed to join at Blair's
Ford, but there was an unforeseen delay. Tarleton was
himself laid by the heels with a violent fever, and it was
some time before he was again in the saddle.

On September 22 Cornwallis wrote piteously to Clinton from his camp at Wacsaw:

If nothing material happens to obstruct my plan of operations, I
mean, as soon as Lieutenant-colonel Tarleton can be removed, to
proceed . . . to Charlotte town, and leave the 71st here until the
sick can be brought on to us. I then mean to make some redoubts,
and establish a fixed post at that place, and to give the command
of it to Major Wemyss, whose regiment is so totally demolished by
sickness, that it will not be fit for actual service for some months.

On the following day Tarleton had recovered sufficiently to travel on a litter. The British army thereupon
moved on to Charlotte.

At this juncture there were further complications. After leaving Camden, Cornwallis had sent orders to Major Patrick Ferguson to join the main army at Charlotte. Although Ferguson for some months had been harassing the upcountry rebels, he had influenced many people but had gained no friends by so doing. On a flat-topped eminence known as King's Mountain in North Carolina, Ferguson was killed, and his force of American Tories was enthusiastically slaughtered by a competent collection of backwoodsmen with long memories and long rifles.

This was a major disaster and it gave Cornwallis pause. He was now compelled to take stock of the weakness of his own army, the extent and poverty of North Carolina and the ruin of his militia.

There appeared to be no alternative. He decided on an abrupt about-face, and as a result His Majesty's troops left Charlotte in a hurry on the evening of October 14. It was a miserable retreat. Either by error or by misunderstanding, the rear guard destroyed the baggage. Thereupon it rained incessantly and the roads were paved with bottomless mud. During the day the hapless soldiers lived on corn from the nearby fields. After long and fatiguing marches, they lay down on the wet ground, missing the tents and the rest of the equipment that had been burned so casually at Charlotte. When the royal forces eventually arrived at the Catawba settlement, the march was now to be delayed for two days more. Not only were the troops ill, a circumstance easily understood, but of all persons, Cornwallis himself was suddenly attacked by a dangerous fever. The command devolved on Rawdon, who successfully kept the forces intact, but it was nearly a month before the earl was again in command and the army garrisoned at Wynnesborough in South Carolina.

As winter set in, the situation on both sides had changed. On the one hand, Nathanael Greene had been given command of the American forces, and although, as he said when he first viewed his new responsibility, "The appearance of the troops was wretched beyond description," he proceeded to plan a campaign. Cornwallis, on the other hand, not only had received reinforcements from England but his troops had regained their health with the advent of colder weather. Despite the fact that the British now considerably outnumbered the tattered rebel army, the noble earl was worried. Much to the amazement of the British commander, Greene had divided his force, placing part of it under the command of Brigadier General Daniel Morgan. Such a move is not the classic procedure ordinarily taken by the commander of the inferior of two opposing forces. Cornwallis, who realized that Greene was no fool, got the point. The Americans, in two divisions, could now live more easily on the countryside. The earl had used that tactic himself in this barren terrain. The strictly military implications did not escape him, either. If he should proceed toward one of the American forces, the other would be free to strike at Ninety-six and Augusta; if he moved toward the second, the first would have a clear road to Charleston. In unorthodox warfare Cornwallis was fully capable of throwing away the rule book himself. He divided his own army into three parts. One, under General Leslie, was to hold Camden against attack. Tarleton was given the assignment of finding and crushing Morgan. Cornwallis would take the remainder of the army into North Carolina and mop up what was left of Morgan's force after Tarleton had put them to flight.

It was magnificent strategy—and the best laid plans went agley at Cowpens. Morgan has been criticized for his choice of battleground, and the disposition of his troops was unorthodox to say the least; but he drove the British from the field, and tarnished forever the reputation of the hitherto unvanquished Banastre Tarleton.

Morgan, however, was cagey enough to realize that he might still be in danger from Cornwallis, so instead of falling back to the north, he went east. Cornwallis, stung by the defeat of his favorite lieutenant and eager to pursue Morgan, spent two days destroying his superfluous baggage. He set a prime example for his army by drastically reducing his own equipment. Wagons and their contents were burned on the spot; and the only ones saved were the vehicles needed to carry ammunition, salt, hospital stores, and four others spared for the transport of the sick and wounded. Otherwise, all was destroyed. The tents went into the fire, the provisions went up in smoke, and most agonizing of all, the rum casks were stove in.

This was far too much for some of the foot soldiers, both Hessian and British. After all, from the point of view of the foreign professional soldier, some of the more delicate ideological nuances involved in this particular conflict were a bit difficult to comprehend. Discomfort and danger he could expect. That was the lot of the soldier anywhere. But insufficient food and no rum? What a war! Better to go over the hill, and so when darkness came, he did in large numbers.

As soon as Greene learned that Cornwallis had destroyed his baggage but was apparently still determined to move north, the wily Quaker was exultant. Greene's idea was to retreat to Virginia, just fast enough to make Cornwallis anxious to follow, but not slow enough to be caught. Greene would be getting closer to his supplies and reinforcements, and the king's army, which had destroyed its stores to gain mobility, would be getting farther from theirs. Morgan disagreed violently with this scheme, but he was now afflicted with the ague, and it is difficult to argue a tactical point during a malarial chill. Morgan then retired from military service for the rest of his life. It was in this fashion that began the famous Retreat to the Dan. After the Catawba was behind both forces, there were still three unbridged rivers to cross, besides innumerable tributaries. There was the Yadkin, the Deep River, and finally the Dan. At any of these, high water or lack of boats might hold up the pursued and force a battle, or hold up the pursuer and let the foe escape. Once across the Dan, Greene would be able to call on reinforcements and supplies and pounce on the exhausted and overextended British.

Greene won the race across the Dan. When Cornwallis arrived on the south bank, he found that the American rear guard had crossed the night before. The river was too high to cross without boats, and Greene had all the boats on the other side. Yet, although Cornwallis may have lost the race, he still had succeeded in chasing the rebels out of the Carolinas. The southern colonies were now firmly in the possession of the King. Even so, it was an empty victory. What could he do now? He could not follow the Americans into Virginia. With nothing more than occasional brushes with the rebels on his way north, Cornwallis had lost 250 men by sickness and desertion on this march. He could not stay here on the south bank of the Dan. His base was well over two hundred long and troublesome miles behind him. There was nothing else to do but turn back. Cornwallis in chagrin returned to Hillsboro.

If the British were in a dilemma, so was Greene. He had allowed himself to be chased all the way back to Virginia, with the idea that there he would have Cornwallis weakened at the end of a supply line. But it was also part of the plan that the American forces would be supplied and reinforced from Virginia. He would then have Cornwallis in a box. The sad realities of the matter were that Greene's reinforcements were not available, and furthermore they might not be for several weeks. His grand opportunity to draw Cornwallis into a trap had faded, and now the Noble Earl, as Cornwallis was nicknamed, was escaping southward again. Greene had saved his little army, but he had failed to maintain American prestige in the Carolinas. Now, in this weird turn of events, there was nothing he could do but chase Cornwallis back into North Carolina. Chase him then he would, but not fast enough to catch him at the wrong place.

There was much maneuvering on both sides. While this was taking place, Greene finally obtained his reinforcements and in mid-March went into camp near Guilford Court House. Cornwallis was short on supplies and in a quandary. Either he had to fight immediately or retreat to the seacoast. It took little time for the earl to make up his mind. He was a fighter, and he was weary of retreats. In the evening of March 14th, he sent off what little remained of his heavy equipment and started for Guilford.

According to the score cards the battle of Guilford Court House was a fairly clear-cut victory for the king's men. They held the field and the Americans retreated. Of about 1,900 men who entered the conflict on the British side, 93 were killed and 493 wounded, so that well over one-fourth of the combatants were casualties. Greene had a considerably larger force, many of whom were untrained militia, but he had less than half as many casualties. Greene had determined not to destroy his army in order to win one battle. Cornwallis had won another engagement, but he realized full well that one more such brilliant victory would so reduce his combat potential that the watchful local patriots would cheerfully come off their farms and out of the swamps and tear him to pieces in an afternoon. His dilemma had merely been compounded by his success.

The earl headed immediately for Cross Creek, a settlement of rigidly loyal Scottish Highlanders on the Cape Fear River. Loyalty alone, even though a valued characteristic, was not enough to feed an army. He desperately needed supplies simply not available at Cross Creek. He had to push on another hundred miles to the coast where he arrived after a melancholy journey interrupted several times for the burial of valued officers dying of their wounds.

On April 7, he was at Wilmington and three days later wrote, somewhat lugubriously, to Clinton:

> I am now employed in disposing of the sick and wounded, and in procuring supplies of all kinds, to put the troops into a proper state to take the field. I am, likewise, impatiently looking out for the expected reinforcement from Europe, part of which will be indispensably necessary to enable me either to act offensively, or even to maintain myself in the upper parts of the country, where alone I can hope to preserve the troops from the fatal sickness which so nearly ruined the army last autumn.

Apparently the Noble Earl was learning some basic facts of military hygiene, but learning them the hard way.

His winter campaign had been rough as well. Between January 15 and April 1, 1781, the troops under his command had dwindled from 3,224 present and fit for duty to 1,723. By the first of May the number was down to 1,435.

While the British commander was pondering his next move, word reached him that Greene had marched south, apparently to attack Rawdon at Camden. Cornwallis was not at all willing to pursue his adversary in that direction. Forage was scanty, and more important, Greene might trap him among the great rivers. Rawdon would have to take care of himself. He notified Germain in London, "I have . . . resolved to take advantage of General Greene's having left the back part of Virginia open, and march immediately into that province to attempt a junction with General Phillips."

Perhaps it was an ill omen, but at this point his principal subordinate, Major General Leslie, was advised by his physicians, because of the serious deterioration of his health, to return to a latitude colder than the Carolinas or Virginia. Leslie thereupon prepared to depart for New York. At about the same time two of his most capable combat captains were attacked by fevers and died.

During the previous December, Benedict Arnold, by now a brigadier general in the British army, had been sent to the Chesapeake area with 1,800 men to annoy enemy communications, destroy stores and supplies that might be useful especially to the southern army, and establish a small naval base for frigates on short raiding expeditions. In March, 1781, Clinton had sent Major General Phillips and a detachment of 2,000 men—"the elite of my army," Sir Henry called them—with directions to take Arnold's contingent under his orders. This combined force would then lie directly across the supply line of Nathanael Greene, whose communications were, of necessity, entirely by land, and would not only interfere with his materiel, but conceivably might provide some diversionary aid to

Cornwallis. The action in Virginia in the early months of
the year, however, consisted primarily in the destruction of
shipyards, vessels, warehouses and arms, all essential to
warfare on the part of the rebels.

Not long after Arnold and Phillips had joined forces,
the latter received word from Cornwallis that he was coming north and would meet him in Petersburg. Phillips, who
had been on his way to Portsmouth, turned back to Petersburg and established himself there to await the arrival of
his superior. On the tenth of May General Phillips was
suddenly taken ill with a high fever, and on the fifteenth
he was dead. So Cornwallis came north. Behind him was a
situation he was eager to avoid. Ahead of him he would
find some useful troops, but a valued lieutenant and friend
would be occupying a grave less than a week old.

In New York, in that spring of 1781, the news of the
self-made decision on the part of Cornwallis to abandon
the struggle in the deep South and move into the Virginia
theater on a mission of conquest was the source of absolute
dismay. Clinton, much to his disgust, was scarcely in a
position to countermand the order. For one thing, communications were faulty and slow, and Cornwallis was
already in Virginia by the time the news of his plans
reached New York. Furthermore, Clinton was so completely frustrated in his attempts to deal with the Royal
Navy in the person of Admiral Arbuthnot that he was
repeatedly offering to resign his command. If the ministry
should accept his resignation, the obvious candidate for
supreme commander would be Cornwallis.

Even though Clinton was in an administrative bind,
his deepest concern was for the awesome aspects of military medicine which he foresaw. "Lord Cornwallis' plan
. . . appears to have been to evacuate New York . . . and
remove the whole army from thence to the sickly province
of Virginia." But even more bitterly did the commander-in-
chief view the timing of the move. "For the commence-
ment of this grand effort His Lordship had selected the
month of June, a period when the deadly epidemics of that

sickly climate begin to rage and all military enterprise ought, of course, to cease, as General Washington repeatedly declares. . . ." There is something about the way he calls as witness his principal military adversary that adds poignancy to Sir Henry's despair.

In the meantime, the rebels and their allies had been active. It was no secret that Washington and Rochambeau had been in conference at Wethersfield, and obviously a joint effort was under consideration. Clinton realized that either he or Cornwallis would probably be under combined attack. Sir Henry felt it imperative to hold New York at all cost. In that case Cornwallis must either use his present strength to divert the enemy from New York, or confine himself to a defensive post and return some of his troops to Clinton.

The importance of a base in Virginia was that an army there could be supported by waterborne communications. The British were dominant at sea, but a base in the area was essential to control the great bay. Cornwallis decided that Portsmouth could not protect ships of the line and furthermore was very unhealthy in warm weather. Yorktown was finally chosen, but the earl, who seems to have had no offensive strategy in mind other than, with more help from New York, to chase Lafayette out of Richmond, was unhappy. He griped to headquarters, "I must again take the liberty of calling Your Excellency's serious attention to the question of the utility of a defensive post in this country, which cannot have the smallest influence on the war in Carolina, and which only gives us some acres of an unhealthy swamp and is forever liable to become the prey of a foreign enemy with a temporary superiority at sea."

From the tactical point of view the early weeks of the summer were on the whole profitless for both sides. The Americans, under Lafayette, were outnumbered, and the wily marquis spent much of his time avoiding a showdown, which at that moment could only have been disastrous. British action during the interval consisted largely of a series of raids on colonists' property, both commercial and military. Much of this was put to the torch, although the efficacy of these sorties was questioned by Tarleton himself. "The stores destroyed, either of a public or private nature, were not in quantity or value equivalent to the damage sustained in the skirmishes on route, and the loss of men and horses by the excessive heat of the climate."

On the fourteenth of August Washington received word that the French fleet under the command of Admiral de Grasse, which had arrived in the Caribbean some weeks earlier, was heading for Chesapeake Bay. Six days later the American and French allies began crossing the Hudson River at King's Ferry. At this time Clinton supposed they were heading for Staten Island to attack him, but it soon became apparent they were heading for Virginia.

In addition to the fleet coming north from the Caribbean, the French had eight ships of the line under Admiral de Barras stationed at Newport. When the Rhode Island squadron sailed for the Chesapeake, a combined British fleet under Admirals Hood and Graves left New York to intercept de Barras. The British were too late, and discovered, on their arrival, that de Grasse was at anchor inside the mouth of the bay.

De Grasse came out to meet the British, and in the late afternoon of the fifth of September a confrontation occurred that Graves described as "a pretty sharp brush" and Mahan considered one of the most significant naval battles in world history. In any case, when the two fleets finally separated, the British had had somewhat the worse of the affair; and after some days of maneuvering returned to New York, whereupon the combined French fleets bottled up Chesapeake Bay.

It would be well at this point to turn our attention to New York. The two previous autumns, those of 1779 and 1780, had been noteworthy because of an unusually heavy prevalence of malaria, both among military personnel and civilians. On August 19 of 1781 Bauermeister wrote cheerfully to his Hessian employer, "The islands of New York are in a redoubtable state of defense; besides, the rebels have made no preparation for an offensive. We are completely inactive. The summer is mild, and the troops as a whole have never been so well as they are now."

Literally, the tune was to change overnight. On the following day Washington was marching south, two and a half weeks later the Battle of the Virginia Capes took place, and on September 12, less than a month after Bauermeister's ebullient letter and a week before the British fleet floundered back into New York harbor, one of the Hessians stationed at Fort Knyphausen noted in his journal, "Our duty here changed from day to day and was very severe, and fevers commenced."

The Battle of the Capes occurred on September 5 and Cornwallis surrendered on October 19. It seems curious that there should have been a delay of six weeks between these events, or at least a delay of a month between the time the fleet finally returned to New York on September 19 and when it finally sailed to the rescue.

Certainly the delay was not solely to await the arrival of reinforcements from Admiral Digby, because he was in New York on the twenty-fourth of September. Even before that, on September 21 Graves wrote to Clinton, ". . . as soon as the fleet can be got into a state for action, I am ready to undertake any service in conjunction with the army that shall be thought advisable." He added, somewhat down in the mouth, that it was quite uncertain when the fleet could be got to sea.

Unquestionably New York was concerned. On September 6 Clinton wrote with considerable understanding to his fellow land officer the Earl Cornwallis that de Grasse had gotten into the Chesapeake and that General Washington was moving against the Virginia post with at least six thousand French and rebel troops, and then continued, "I think the best way to relieve you, is to join you, as soon as possible, with all the force that can be spared from hence, which is about four thousand men. They are already embarked, and will proceed the instant I receive information from the Admiral that we may venture. . . ."

There was a great deal of activity in New York during this interlude. According to Bauermeister:

> Since the 6th of this month [September] all the grenadiers of the army, the 22nd, 37th, 42nd, and 57th Regiments, the Leib Regiment, and Prinz Carl's have been embarked. But on the 19th all these disembarked again on Staten Island, and by this time (Sept. 24) everything has been brought ashore. Sickness is increasing. Until Admiral Graves's fleet is reinforced, no ships can leave this harbor. . . . At present it looks very bad for Lord Cornwallis's army. . . . The Hesse-Hanau Free Corps has been moved from Flushing to Brooklyn, since more than half of them are ill and forty-six men and one officer have died.

On the very same day Clinton was reassuring Cornwallis, ". . . it is determined, that above five thousand men, rank and file, shall be embarked on the King's ships and the joint exertions of the navy and army made in a few days to relieve you, and afterwards co-operate with you. . . . There is every reason to hope we start from hence the 5th October." But they did not start by the fifth, and how much of the delay was due to disease is impossible to say. On October 16, the day before the rescue mission did actually put to sea, Bauermeister, in contrast to his recent enthusiasm, was writing:

> Bilious fever and ague are very common; the hospitals are filling up, and great numbers are dying. The approaching cold weather, it is hoped, will do more for the sick than all the nursing and medicine, for these unavoidable diseases on these islands are due to the change from summer to fall.

This etiologic note by a layman would scarcely have been contradicted by any medical officer in His Majesty's service at the time. In this connection, Admiral Graves wrote a peculiar note to Clinton on October 17, the day he sailed to relieve the besieged at Yorktown.

> There has, I hope, been no mistake. For, as we cannot sail until about ten o'clock this forenoon, and can then go but little below Denyses, I would not give you unnecessary alarm; and meant to have sent an officer at eight o'clock, when I would have explained to Your Excellency that all this show of signals and topsails were

no other than so many spurs to push forward the lazy and supine. And I am sorry to find that *difficulties go on increasing, and that nothing can turn the current* but being actually at sea.

This is indeed a strange comment to come from the pen of an admiral of His Majesty's navy. One cannot belp wonder if "the lazy and supine" were suffering from chills and fever, especially since a sea voyage might hopefully be curative. This, however, is mere speculation.

As the summer waned, Cornwallis at Yorktown was in trouble. In August he wrote, ". . . the fatigue and difficulty of constructing works in this warm season, convinces me, that all the labour that the troops here will be capable of, without ruining their health, will be required at least for six weeks to put the intended works in this place in a tolerable state of defense."

On September 8 he reported, "The army is not very sickly. Provisions for six weeks . . . I will be very careful of it."

But nine days later there was an ominous note, "This place is in no state of defense. If you cannot relieve me very soon, you must be prepared to hear the worst."

And then on September 29th, "I shall retire this night within the works . . . Medicines are wanted."

Medicines are wanted. It is a plaintive, pitiful cry. It is a heart-rending appeal that has gone out in every generation from every part of the world. It is the cry of the city that is besieged, of the soldier bivouacked in the swamp, of the sailor whose mouth is filled with blood. The want of medicine would once again affect the political history of a nation, for when the surrender took place at Yorktown, about one-third of the besieged troops were ill—too ill to be effective—and most of them ill from malaria.

The mosquito, of course, has no political or military motivations, nor does it show partisanship in the disputes of man. Americans and their French allies were attacked frequently and often severely by the same insect assailants. Some of the Americans, however, had lived in endemic areas and had a degree of immunity denied their enemies; also their recruits were not three thousand miles away. The French, on the other hand, were not importantly involved in many campaigns where much marching, fighting, and temporary bivouacs were necessary. Certainly the British and German troops were more frequently exposed and more seriously attacked by the disease. Furthermore, their therapy was not always of the best even when available. According to Dr. Jackson:

> The Hessians were all of them inveterate enemies to the bark; and there were ever some of the British surgeons who employed it very sparingly. The mortality among the troops trusted to the care of those, was uniformly in great proportion. There was a Hessian regiment, the situation of which I had the opportunity of knowing exactly, that lost one third of its men by this disease and its effects, during one year's service in Georgia. There were British regiments also, which lost more than a fourth; while there were others, which did not lose a twentieth. The whole of these regiments were engaged on the same services; they were all alike foreigners in America; and there appeared to be no obvious cause for so great a difference in the degree of mortality, except a difference in the management of the bark. . . .

But mortality figures by no means are the most important measure of the significance of malaria. Although a sick soldier may recover to fight again, during a campaign he is no more effective than a dead one, and temporarily, at least, is more of a nuisance. He ties up the attentions of others to take care of him and to furnish him transportation. Illness also was no respecter of rank. Before the war was over Rawdon went back to England, shattered in health, and General Leslie and Brigadier General Patterson had to leave the theater of operation for the same reason. At a crucial point in the southern campaign Tarleton was laid by the heels, and shortly thereafter Cornwallis was disabled by a fever, and General Phillips died of a febrile illness.

So, on the long, long road that ultimately lead to Yorktown, there was malaria in the West Indies, malaria in Florida and along the Gulf of Mexico, malaria in Georgia, malaria in the Carolinas, malaria in Virginia and in New York. There can be little doubt that General Washington at Yorktown had, in addition to the French forces commanded by de Grasse, Rochambeau, and Lafayette, another ally—unhonored, unsung, unrecognized—but at least equally potent and fully as effective. This was the *Anopheles* mosquito.

5

The Fleet That Failed

It was autumn 1778, and the young Marquis de Lafayette was ready for a vacation. For more than a year he had been in the thick of revolutionary events, but here in America there would be little military activity during the approaching winter. Armies on foot, on horseback, or dependent on wagon trains had little maneuverability where roads were clogged with snow, bridges were far apart, and rivers were coated with treacherous ice.

There were compelling reasons for a trip to Europe at this time. During the interval since his farewell to his young wife, Adrienne had given birth to a second daughter and in solitude had mourned the death of their first. Furthermore, perhaps by personal contact he might persuade the French ministry to send a sizeable land force to aid the colonial rebellion.

Although the thought was neither expressed nor implied, General Washington contemplated the temporary departure of his eager aide with a certain sense of relief. For a few months at least Lafayette's energy and enthusiasm would not be missed. There were many matters requiring sober and uninterrupted reflection on the part of the commander-in-chief.

The original idea was for Lafayette to return to France in one of the ships of the fleet of Admiral d'Estaing. This was the French naval force of twelve ships of the line and five frigates that had sailed from Toulon the previous April. The fleet was intended to cross the Atlantic and blockade the British Admiral Howe in Delaware Bay, thus preventing General Clinton from evacuating Philadelphia easily and establishing himself in New York. The idea was excellent, but the French dragged their keels. It took them a month to pass Gibraltar, and when they appeared off the Delaware capes on the seventh of July, Howe's fleet had gone. The British army, having chosen to travel overland, after struggling with Washington's colonials and the hideous heat of the Jersey flatlands, was already in New York.

The subsequent career of d'Estaing's force was similarly undistinguished. When he returned to seek out Howe he had been unable to find pilots who would guide his heavy-draft ships over the bar into New York. After some eleven days of maneuvering he sailed for Newport, but again luck was against him. Misunderstandings beset his relationships with the American General Sullivan on land, and heavy weather broke up his attempt to do battle with the British at sea. Because of serious damage to his ships from a fierce August storm, he put into Boston for repairs. After some uncomfortable weeks there, he sailed on November 4 for the West Indies without bothering to let his American allies know his destination.

Meanwhile, Congress, eager to demonstrate its gratitude toward Lafayette, suggested that a new American vessel, due to sail from Boston, should carry the nobleman home. Late in October the marquis mounted his horse in Philadelphia and with a few companions began the long ride to Massachusetts. It was a cold, wet, tedious journey. The horses bore up well, but the riders suffered. By the time the travelers had reached Fishkill on the Hudson, Lafayette had developed what appears to have been a severe pneumonia. He remained at Fishkill for some weeks, during which time General Washington rode over from headquarters to make frequent visits. The general sent Dr. John Cochran, who bore the awesome title of physician and surgeon general of the middle department of the army, to attend the marquis and accompany him to Boston, where the invalid's convalescence was reportedly hastened with the help of good Madeira wine.

At Boston there were further delays. The new frigate of thirty-six guns, appropriately christened the *Alliance,* had been built at Salisbury Point on the Merrimac, and was seaworthy. Signing on a crew, however, was no easy matter. This was wartime, but there was no navy and therefore no dockside personnel with either military experience or patriotic motivation. Seamen were not readily available on the New England coast to sail on such a voyage. This was no privateer, with the possibility of plunder and profit. On the other hand it was an armed vessel about to sail alone through hostile waters, carrying a passenger the enemy would be delighted to seize.

At this turn of events the Massachusetts council was embarrassed and offered to resort to press gangs in order to recruit a crew. To Lafayette, already becoming a symbol of freedom, this was scarcely fitting, so that idea was promptly abandoned. The alternative finally chosen was hardly an improvement. At last a motley mob of convicts and a collection of deserters from the British army were assembled to form a crew. At least, as a later generation would say, they were warm bodies. Finally on January 11, 1779, the *Alliance* cleared from Boston.

It was a miserable trip. The North Atlantic seas were rough and the winter gales carried away her topmasts by the time the ship was off the Newfoundland banks. The vessel sprang a leak and, tossed about by furious storms, high winds and huge waves, there were many long, fearsome nights when all on board expected the *Alliance* to founder on her maiden voyage. But gradually the ship approached the waters closer to Europe, the weather improved, the passengers relaxed. France was only a few hundred miles away.

Even so there was more trouble ahead. One calm day when the officers were at dinner an American seaman insisted on speaking to Lafayette on an urgent matter. A short time before this ship had left Boston a proclamation had been issued by George III encouraging the crews of rebel vessels to mutiny. They could then seize their ships and sail them to England where they could be sold as prizes, the spoils being divided among the mutineers. The cutthroats and criminals manning the *Alliance* were plotting to seize control that very afternoon and steer for an English port where the Marquis would doubtless bring a high price on delivery. It was all very carefully planned. Someone topside would cry, "A sail." When the officers rushed on deck to view the stranger they would be immediately overpowered by the mutinous crew.

That was the scheme, but as soon as Lafayette and his friends were apprised of it they went into action. The loyal French and Americans were assembled and the officers went below decks where the watch still slept, dreaming of riches that would soon be theirs. With a few swift sword strokes the hammock cords of the ringleaders were cut, and before they could disentangle themselves from cordage and surprise they were clapped in irons and finished the voyage in the brig.

The marquis landed at Brest on February 6, took a post chaise and arrived at Versailles on the twelfth. He found that France was bristling with plans and action. Ever since the Peace of Paris a decade and a half before there had been many in France with a burning urge to avenge that disgrace and the loss of Canada. When the Americans defeated Burgoyne at Saratoga, the French had been convinced that they now had an opportunity as well as an excuse to declare war on England. Furthermore, negotiations were under way which shortly would bring Spain, eager to get back Gibraltar and Florida, into the hostilities as an ally of France. There was to be an invasion of England that summer.

Lafayette was agog. In his own words the idea made him "tremble with joy." He and Benjamin Franklin discussed plans for an amphibious assault on a major seaport such as Liverpool, the marquis to be in charge of the troops and John Paul Jones commanding the naval task force.

Somehow the scheme leaked out and the city of Liverpool, considering itself defenseless, was terrified, but neither the French king nor the ministry was impressed. This onslaught was to be no mere raid, conducted by adventurers and boys, but rather a full-scale, two-nation military offensive, organized, equipped, and conducted by experienced professionals. Sartine, the French Minister of Marine was assigned the task of fitting out the expedition. Admiral d'Orvilliers, who had had an indecisive brush with the British Admiral Keppel off Ushant the previous July, was in command of the French naval force. Admiral Don Luis de Cordova was the Spanish fleet commander. The French army of invasion was headed by the Comte de Vaux whose military success against General Paoli some years before had resulted in the annexation of Corsica to France. The feeling was if de Vaux could conquer one island why not another?

The mounting offensive potential of the allies appeared more formidable with every passing day. By the end of May, 50,000 well equipped and well trained French soldiers had been collected at Le Havre and St. Malo. Morale was high among the officers, and highest of all in the Quarter-Master General, the Marquis de Lafayette. In addition, some 400 transports had been gathered along the French coast to move this huge army across the Channel as soon as the waters had been safely cleared of the British fleet.

At this point France had about eighty ships of the line in good condition and some 67,000 seamen on duty. Spain had about sixty ships of the line, and the British admitted that the allied vessels were superior in size and in artillery to their own.

The British fleet was scattered, and by stern necessity. Many of its fighting ships, large and small, were patrolling the coastline of North America from the St. Lawrence to the Chesapeake. The experience of Burgoyne at Saratoga, moreover, had demonstrated to London that military action against the rebels could be hazardous if unsupported by strength at sea. So large a segment of the navy had been committed to the colonial revolt that the Channel fleet was reduced to about forty ships of the line.

But British naval impotence at this juncture was by no means solely due to dispersion of her fighting ships. Corruption and intrigue at the highest levels of government was rife, particularly involving Lord Sandwich, the First Lord of the Admiralty. Following the Battle of Ushant in July 1778, Admiral Keppel was court-martialed. The charges were generally thought to be trumped up and politically motivated. Although he was acquitted with honor, the anger and discontent in the upper echelons of the navy were so great that twenty of the highest ranking officers were on the verge of resigning their commissions. They were argued out of this action by their friends, but the admiralty was in such straits that the command of the Channel fleet was finally given to Sir Charles Hardy, dragged out of retirement, considered incompetent by his juniors, and at the age of sixty-three generally regarded as old for his years and physically unfit for such grave responsibility.

Meanwhile the King of Spain was in a frenzy. Once the decision for invasion had been made, immediate action was mandatory. The strategy called for the French and Spanish fleets to join off the coast of Spain near Corunna and sail for the English Channel. There they would clean out the British defenders, whereupon the troop transports, waiting on the Normandy and Brittany coasts, would then be able to cross unopposed.

Because of Spanish insistence on hurried departures, d'Orvilliers sailed from Brest on June 3, his ships inadequately manned and with insufficient supplies for a long expedition. One item did come aboard in oversupply. Well over a century later it would be identified and named *Rickettsia prowazeki,* the causative organism of typhus fever.

Typhus fever has a long and significant history in the annals of disease and war. Dr. Hans Zinsser in his classic

biography of typhus, *Rats, Lice and History*, believes that
it began to appear in a recognizable form in the sixteenth
century, but it was not until well into the twentieth that its
etiology and mode of transmission were worked out. Tech-
nically, rickettsiae of which there are several known species and which in turn are responsible for several diseases,
are neither bacteria nor viruses, but they have some of the
characteristics of both.

Rickettsia prowazeki is transmitted to man by the bite
of the body louse. The organism shortly appears in the
blood stream and sets up a violent reaction, accompanied
by high fever, headache, bodily aches and pains, and a skin
rash. The acute phase often lasts for two weeks, and the
mortality may run as high as twenty percent. In epidemic
form the disease has been known by a variety of names,
including putrid fever, from its obvious association with
filth; and war fever, camp fever, ship fever, and jail fever
among others. Although the connection went unrecognized for centuries, these were the commonest places
where men and lice were intimately crowded together.

The French appeared at the agreed rendezvous on
June 11, but many of the Spaniards had been in much less
of a hurry than their king. Long sultry days dragged by
with no sign of the allies. On the second of July the Ferrol
division of the Spanish navy arrived, but it was a full three
more sweltering weeks before the main body from Cadiz
under de Cordova appeared. At this point it was suddenly
discovered that the two allies could not understand each
other's signals, so several more days elapsed while signal
books were translated and agreements reached on sailing
orders.

By this time the close association of lice and men, the
utter disregard of sanitation and the summer heat had
created the ideal atmosphere for typhus. The French
found it necessary to put 500 of their sickest men ashore at
Corunna, but 2000 more who were feverish were kept
aboard when the combined fleets finally hoisted anchor on
July 30 and headed north.

The armament that now bore down on the English Channel was the greatest naval force that had ever been seen afloat. Sixty-six ships of the line and fourteen frigates drove for the poorly protected coast of Britain. As they sailed in double column they covered four and a half miles of sea. But the strength of a navy is not solely in ships and guns. Although the more enlightened medical men and line officers in the British navy were beginning to think of disease prevention in terms of cleanliness and attention to diet, such advanced ideas were by no means universally held in that service, and certainly had not penetrated to the continent. It would be difficult to imagine a more favorable milieu for the rapid spread of infectious disease than a French battleship of the eighteenth century. A hulk whose dimensions were 170 by 50 feet might carry 1000 men or more. On this expedition the food was poor to begin with and had ample opportunity to spoil. The water was dirty and in short supply. The summer heat was terrific. The portholes were blocked by cannon. The hammocks were hung so close together and so near to the undersurface of the deck that it was actually a struggle to get into them. Many of the ships carried no one with any medical training, and others lacked even a medical chest.

The allies entered the Channel without sighting Hardy, who at that moment was cruising west of the Scilly Islands off the Cornwall coast. On the sixteenth of August the French admiral wrote to his ministry: "The combined fleet is at this moment becalmed and anchored in sight of the Tower of Plymouth. . . . The situation of the French ships, of which I have already informed you, becomes worse every day, both because of sickness which is prevalent and because of the small quantity of water and provisions with which they are provided."

That same day d'Orvilliers was notified that a supply convoy would soon sail from Brest to come to his aid, but again the timing was poor. Although the general in command of Plymouth later commented that his defenses had been so completely neglected by the British government that the dockyard could have been taken in six hours, the allies had dawdled too long. On the seventeenth the calm was shattered by an easterly wind that soon became a gale. Four days later the combined fleet had been blown a hundred miles from Plymouth.

The same gale carried Hardy westward also, and when d'Orvilliers finally learned the location of the British, he called a council of war to determine what to do next. The officers brought grim tidings. Fever was raging in the fleet and fatalities were mounting. Provisions were running short. The decision was to chase Hardy in the open sea rather than to risk maneuvering this unwieldy body of ships again in the Channel with such weakened crews. But Hardy had other ideas. The wily old man eluded the allies and sailed up the Channel himself, where he could now take advantage of what shore batteries were available. He anchored off Plymouth on September 1.

D'Orvilliers then abandoned the pursuit, and the reasons are not hard to discover. From the 100-gun vessel of the Comte de Guichen 60 bodies had been dropped into the sea and 500 more were on the sick list. Another vessel had already had 70 deaths from the pestilence and now listed 600 sick. On board a third ship, carrying a complement of 800 men, only 360 were fit for duty. Nearly every return from all of the ships of the fleet showed 300, or 400 or 500 men excused from duty, and the ghastly death toll continued to rise. One captain reported that he simply did not have enough men to go aloft to make sail, and many were convinced that the most they could do would be to handle their ships, but it would be impossible to maneuver them in battle or man the guns.

Admiral d'Orvilliers now sent eight of his warships, mere floating hospitals, back to France. His own son, a promising young naval officer, had died in the epidemic. Versailles finally recognized that the expedition was hopeless and ordered the fleet back to Brest, where it anchored on September 14. The Spanish then steered for Cadiz, filling their sails with unkind remarks about the French.

But what about Hardy? Historians universally have dealt brutally with him. He was incompetent. He was old and feeble, and actually he did die that following spring. He ran away. First he ran away beyond the Scillies and then he ran away up the Channel. All that could be said in his favor was that he kept his fleet intact in the face of a truly formidable armada nearly twice the size of his own. Nobody seems to have bothered to note whether this much maligned old man, with his forlorn hope of a fleet, might not have had problems other than merely military. Perhaps he did. According to the records of Haslar, the great naval hospital at Portsmouth, Sir Charles unloaded 2,500 cases of typhus fever from his own contingent there in September 1779, but even so he was compelled to carry along with him 1,000 more sick on board because there was not enough room in the hospital for the remainder. Almost the entire crew of the *Intrepid* either died at sea or were sent to the hospital, while in addition the *Canada,* the *Shrewsbury,* the *London* and the *Namur* were forced out of service, so completely were they disabled by fever. Poor Hardy, sneered at and despised by his nation and its historians because he did not blast his enemy from the water, burdened as he was by cargoes of sickly seamen, probably accomplished more by avoiding a battle than he could possibly have gained by winning one.

And so the greatest allied armada of wooden ships ever gathered together went home without firing a shot. For one whole summer the British Isles, already engaged in a global war, were threatened with invasion by a potent fleet, heavily gunned, and backed up by a large land force capable of a disastrous amphibious onslaught. Nothing of the sort occurred, and the principal obstacle was the interference of a tiny organism too small to be seen, and the existence of which no one was aware.

On land during that same summer the enormous energy of Lafayette was still very much in evidence. He had influence at court and was also a confidante of the ministers. Much of his time was spent dashing back and

forth from his designated military post at Le Havre to his
assumed diplomatic post at Versailles. He consulted with
officials. He wrote voluminously—letters, notes, memo-
randa, and reports. He fired off hints and suggestions to
Franklin in Paris and General Washington in America.
And all the while he was waiting for the return of the
triumphant fleet, his vast, potent army of invasion was
literally going down the drain. Dysentery so afflicted the
troops at St. Malo and Le Havre during that long, hot
summer that this magnificent fighting force was destroyed. The entire campaign was now abandoned and
Lafayette wrote to Vergennes, the minister of foreign
affairs, that he could only weep in silence.

His tears were soon dried, however, and his silence
promptly broken. The marquis was busier and more effective than ever. Both Vergennes and the elderly prime
minister, Maurepas, were coming around to realize, after
this debacle, that the only salvation of France would be in a
major military effort on the North American continent. A
fleet and an army would be dispatched to the colonies. In
that sense the disasters of the summer of 1779 were not
wholly in vain. By a devious route they led to Yorktown.

6

Napoleon and the Mosquito

The purchase of the vast Louisiana Territory in 1803 by the fledgling republic of the United States, then in existence less than a decade and a half, is a familiar and oft-told tale. The troubles of the settlers along the Mississippi, the diplomatic maneuverings and the secret treaties perplexing Jefferson, and finally the startling results of the conversations between Monroe and Livingston on the one hand and Talleyrand on the other are now all part of our folklore. The sale had a significant economic and political impact on our growth and development. The deed not only was of the utmost importance to us in our emergence as a world power, but also is one which has received due attention from historians. In spite of the detailed scrutiny of scholars, it is not generally appreciated that, barring certain purely medical circumstances, the Louisiana Territory might never have been ours at all. More effective than the schemings of Pitt, more powerful than the legions of the first consul, more subtle than the diplomacy of Jefferson, was, as it turned out, the utterly dreadful activity of the mosquito.

The conflict that Americans provincially label the French and Indian War was far more extensive than a series of skirmishes among scattered outposts in North America. Britain was also engaged in a titanic struggle against France and later Spain, after the signing of the Family Pact in 1761. Spain's decision to become an ally of

149

France in this particular fracas was an unexcelled example of poor timing. At that exact moment the British navy was more than equal in ships, in guns, and in manpower to the combined fleets of both her enemies. No official hearts sank in London when war between England and Spain was declared in January, 1762.

As a matter of fact, this turn of events fitted in very well with the overall scheme for the enhancement of the British Empire. More than a year earlier, in this same conflict, Canada had already fallen to Wolfe. Now further lush gains loomed. For a long time the covetous eye of Britain had been frequently cast in the direction of Louisiana, and at this moment a splendid opportunity presented itself. With both France and Spain in the opposite corner, British campaign plans for the year 1762 could crystallize. They called, first of all, for the conquest of Martinique, the French headquarters in the Windward Islands. The next move would be the capture of Havana, guaranteeing control of the rich island of Cuba and incidentally lessening, for future exploitation, the resistance of St. Domingo and Panama. Finally, there would be a powerful blow at Louisiana, which would completely banish the French from North America and at the same stroke give Britain overwhelming dominance on this continent.

On paper this rather elaborate campaign was fleshed out with sixteen thousand troops. Lord Albemarle was given the supreme command and assigned four thousand men to sail with him from England. These were to be united with eight thousand who were already in the West Indies under Monckton. In addition four thousand more were to be recruited in the American colonies by Sir Jeffrey Amherst and sent down to join the tropical festivities.

London had instructed Albemarle most carefully as to his behavior. As soon as the Havana expedition "had had its issue," General Amherst was to take the colonial troops and enough more to make up a force of eight thousand and proceed against French Louisiana. Amherst's intentions, however, were by no means to confine his activities to the area around New Orleans. This, from his point of view, was to be an all-out affair. The Illinois country, in fact all of the northern part of the territory, was to be seized. The prize was all of French North America.

The results were somewhat different than had been anticipated. Martinique, as it turned out, was no problem. Monckton had it when Albemarle landed, but it had been obtained at a considerable and somewhat disheartening cost. The new commander found on his arrival in the West Indies, much to his dismay, what he described as "the remains of a very fine army," reduced not by battle casualties but by sickness. He was able to assemble about twelve thousand men, of whom more than twelve hundred were sick. The type of illness suffered by the troops at that particular time cannot be readily diagnosed at present. Certainly a high proportion of it, however, was malaria.

The provincial forces from North America had not yet arrived, nor did they, as a matter of fact, until the campaign was nearly concluded. In spite of this, the military exigencies of the situation did not allow sufficient time for the invalids to recover. The expedition sailed, therefore, with the men available and landed a little north of the city of Havana on the seventh of June.

Fighting in the tropics, especially the wet tropics, is hell for any troops at any time. Only mad dogs and Englishmen would have tackled Cuba in June, but a fortuitous circumstance added immeasurably to the miseries and fatalities of the British at Havana.

Two years earlier a new governor for Cuba was being readied in Madrid for his colonial assignment. He had been informed by the king that the recent attitude of Britain had appeared to be definitely hostile, and that it would be his duty, as governor, to prepare the defenses of the island against possible attack.

Because of this intelligence, the new official, after his arrival in Havana early in 1761, began constructing new quarters for soldiers and also started work on the fortifications of Cabanas, a hill near the Morro Castle guarding the entrance to the harbor. The labor force for this work was recruited from among the slaves in Vera Cruz. When the slaves arrived, they did not come alone.

For more than a hundred years, since 1655 in fact, there had been no yellow fever in Cuba. It had died out, as it does when the delicate balance of biological requisites is not met, and it now was reintroduced by the slaves whose efforts were to aid in the defense of the city. The arrival of the infection was just in time to hamper the Spaniards, who were afflicted in great numbers, but also just in time to smite their enemy a fearful blow.

The siege of Havana was rough work. The terrain, the climate and the defenses were all formidable, but worse, far worse than any of these were malaria, dysentery, and above all yellow fever. The heat was terrific, the water was brackish, the swamps were impenetrable, the rations were horrid; and over everything the mosquitoes swarmed.

By the middle of July casualties from disease had already assumed serious proportions; scarcely more than half the men were fit for duty. It was nearly the end of the month before the much needed colonial troops arrived, just about the time the Morro was taken. After that it was only a matter of time, although time was taking a heavy toll on the besiegers. On the tenth of August the Spaniards proposed a capitulation and Albemarle had good reason to be devoutly thankful. His army was literally melting away in the tropical sun. He had one brigade of four battalions that would not muster twenty men fit for duty, and although he hastened to ship it back to America, Amherst could spare him no replacements. The situation in the rest of his command was not much better. The commander fervently hoped that after the utterly exhausting work of the siege was over the health of the army might improve, but such was not to be the case. In spite of better quarters, better rations and more rest, the morbidity rate obstinately climbed.

The losses during the siege actually attributable to enemy fire were 560 from the army and 86 from the navy.

Incidentally, James Lind, the famous surgeon of the British navy, states that in this campaign, of the wounded who had limb amputations, five of every six died of tetanus. The total of killed and wounded was slightly under a thousand, but adding together the army, navy and marine casualties, there were six thousand deaths from disease.

The situation reached such extremes that on October 18 a Spanish official wrote to the minister of war at Madrid, "The extraordinary mortality of the British troops has reduced them to the state which . . . if at this moment eight or ten vessels arrived with two or three thousand men to debark, it would not be forty-eight hours before they would capitulate." But the eight or ten vessels did not arrive and the British had Havana.

But the next move was a different matter. Amherst's high hopes of a major offensive against French Louisiana were dashed by the grim realities that faced him after the tropical victory. When Havana fell, Albemarle, true to his instructions, promptly returned to North America some of the units that had been sent from there to help him. When Amherst hurried to the Port of New York to greet them, he was staggered at the spectacle. Writing to Viscount Ligonier on September 23, he commented ruefully, "These troops are arrived here in such a Deplorable Melancholy State as is not to be conceived without seeing them." In October he noted that Albemarle's regulars had been so decimated by the great mortality that other units he had been hoping to receive were being retained in Cuba to serve as garrison troops. The havoc wrought by yellow fever among the conquerors of Havana rendered utterly impossible the projected assault on Louisiana, and a few months later the peace treaty was signed at Paris.

FROM NATCHEZ TO MOBILE

The Peace of Paris, signed in February, 1763, was enough to make the British soldiers who had died in the mosquito-ridden swamps and on the torrid hillsides of

Havana turn in their shallow, sodden graves. Once again the young men fought the battles and the old men wrote the peace. When it was settled, the British withdrew from Cuba and handed it back to Spain in an exchange for Florida, which at that time included a strip of land along the Gulf of Mexico as far as the Mississippi River.

If the military had any regrets at this outcome of their costly victory, the politicians did not. There was a great deal of smug satisfaction in the British government over this bargain. With a potent base at Pensacola, and another at Mobile, the Gulf would now become a British lake. These fortresses would control the traffic between the Spanish port of New Orleans and Europe. Furthermore, there were great potentialities for the development of the territory. It was accessible from the sea and the hinterland could be approached from the Mississippi and the rivers entering the Mobile Bay. A passage was found, through lakes and bayous, whereby shallow draft vessels could go from the Gulf into the Mississippi, completely bypassing New Orleans. In London the ministry could foresee the growth of a stout new arm of the empire. Colonies would be established, cotton and sugar cane would be cultivated, trade would be developed and sooner or later, the Spaniards could be squeezed out of Louisiana. Obviously, something went wrong, and perhaps the real reason why the schemes and dreams for West Florida went awry has been obscured by more compelling and dramatic events.

In the summer of 1765, Colonel Henry Bouquet, who had acquired justifiable renown by his successes against the Indians in western Pennsylvania during Pontiac's War, was given command of the southern district and arrived at Pensacola to assume his new duties. Ten days later he was dead of a fever, his death an unrecognized omen.

James Lind gives us a valuable side light on what the British were facing in Florida.

> At Pensacola, where the soil is sandy and quite barren, the English have suffered much by sickness; some, for want of vegetables, died of scurvy; but a far greater part of fever. The excessive

heat of the weather has sometimes produced in this place a severe fever, similar to that which in the West Indies goes under the name of yellow fever. This, in the year 1765, proved very fatal to a regiment of soldiers sent from England, unseasoned to such climates, from the unfortunate circumstance of their being landed there in the height of the sickly season. It raged chiefly in the fort, where the air in the soldiers' barracks, being sheltered from the sea-breeze by the walls of the fort, was extremely sultry and unhealthy.

Another historian tells us that, "In the year 1765, a regiment of British troops arrived [at Mobile] from Jamaica, and brought with them a contagious distemper." This, too, was yellow fever which had been absent from these shores for sixty years, and the information we have indicates that this was the only such epidemic to occur during the period now under consideration. It was the final lash of the storm that had devastated the British in Cuba. Apparently their major disease problem after this episode, aside from the usual dysenteries and camp ailments, was malaria.

A Survey of West Florida made in 1768 reveals ample reason for the prevalence of malaria.

Mobile . . . is situated among Swamps and Marshes, by the Side of a slow River, in which the Tide is very small, not rising above two feet, and that only once in twenty four Hours; thus, there is no Stream of Water to give a Current to the Air, which becomes stagnated and corrupt. its great Distance too from the Coast frequently deprives it of the Sea Breezes during the hot season, and even when they do blow, they pass over so many Woods and Marshes, that they become tainted. for all these Reasons it is a most unhealthful Place.

As might be anticipated the reports, particularly from the garrison at Mobile, have a dreadful monotony. In 1767 the commanding general noted that fevers were already prevalent by the end of April. The following year there were fifteen deaths in the month of June alone, and only two officers fit for service. In August the sick were evacuated to Pensacola, where conditions were somewhat better, but four died even on the brief passage.

The next spring the fevers were again raging when the warm days of May arrived, and the grim accounts continue year by year. In August, 1772, the despairing general wrote to his superiors that the whole of the garrison would soon be in hospital.

In England the ministers and the land speculators were wringing their hands. In spite of the effulgent advertisements and the urgings of the government, little interest was shown in the new enterprise. Rumors first, and then cruel facts had found their way home. The soldiers were dying far from any battleground. West Florida was an unhealthy sink, and the English farmers and tradesmen were not enthusiastic about migrating to a subtropical grave.

Along the banks of the Mississippi the situation wasn't quite so bad. Scattered along the river, but mostly clustered around the forts at Manchac near Lake Pontchartrain, at Baton Rouge, and at Natchez, were prosperous colonies. They never grew to any size, and since little has been written about them, we can only speculate as to the reason. Perhaps one inkling might be found in the report, written a generation before, by a Jesuit missionary describing a trip up the Mississippi from New Orleans. It was a hard trip. "But none of these others are worthy to be mentioned with the musketoes. This little insect has caused more swearing since the French have been in Mississippi than had previously taken place in all the rest of the world."

Perhaps during the later period when the English occupied the riparian colonies, the reason they recorded their experiences so sparsely was their frantically flailing quills.

An entirely new situation was now about to be introduced. When the original colonies scattered along the Atlantic seaboard revolted against the mother country in 1776, the English along the river remained loyal to the king, but they were too scattered and too few to make any important contribution to that conflict. From the military point of view, however, the situation now changed. As soon as England realized that a short war was impossible, she also recognized the fact that not only France but Spain would join the enemy. In May, 1779, Spain declared war. This meant that an opportunity had now presented itself for Britain to seize the lands in America still held by the Spanish. The appetite of an empire is never satisfied. An elaborate plan was devised by the war ministry. First, a large party of northwestern Indians was to swoop down on St. Louis; next, an expedition was to set forth from Detroit to invade Kentucky and occupy the attentions of George Rogers Clark; and finally General John Campbell, stationed at Pensacola, would push up the Mississippi with a fleet and an army and unite with the northern expeditions at Natchez. From thence the Illinois country and all the Spanish settlements along the river would be taken. It was a brilliant plan, and if successful, the territory north of the Ohio River might even now be part of the province of Quebec.

The cold military facts of the situation did not warrant any such strategic concepts. The two northern expeditions were entirely feasible, but the task assigned to Campbell was utterly unrealistic unless he were to be given more aid than the circumstances would allow. The military posts on the Gulf that were to serve as his bases were unhealthy and poorly manned. Furthermore they were dependent on the outside world for supplies which could only come by sea, and the Spanish naval base at Havana was five hundred miles nearer to Florida than was Port Royal in Jamaica. Finally, New Orleans was ideally placed to cut off the Mississippi forts.

At this point, the fortunes of war took a hand. The Spaniards in New Orleans learned about the actual declaration of hostilities before the British received the news; so just when Campbell was ready to set out for the conquest of New Orleans, he learned that the feeble forts along the Mississippi had been surprised and captured by the able and energetic young Spanish Governor Galvez.

This was a serious setback, but it was not necessarily fatal. To regain the lost territory, or even to hold what they had, the British needed reinforcements. Clinton had no troops to spare; his own reinforcements that summer had arrived at New York with typhus on board. The troops would have to come from the Caribbean, and there were troubles there. In April of 1779 the general at St. Lucia was reporting to London, "Without bark we should not have a man fit for duty in three months. . . ." That same month, more than one man out of four was on sick report, and there were a hundred deaths. A multitude of similar instances might be cited. Four new regiments arrived at St. Lucia in July of the following year and then sailed to Jamaica. By the time they landed, out of 2,300 men, 168 were dead and 780 on the sick list. During the remainder of that year 1,100 men died in Jamaica alone. There were simply no reinforcements available, and as for Campbell's own situation, he had already reported to Clinton, "Of the troops that now remain under my command, 63 sargeants and 724 rank and file are returned fit for duty. But I can assure Your Excellency that above 100 of these are perfect invalids . . . for only the infirm and unfit for service of the 16th Regiment were left here."

With an aggressive opponent such as Galvez, there could be only one outcome. Mobile was taken in March of 1780 and the following year Pensacola fell to the same capable commander. The British occupation of West Florida and the Mississippi Valley, begun with such confidence less than twenty years before, thus came to an ignominious end. If the English had been successful, the Spaniards and the French would have been out of the area and there would have been no peaceful purchase by the Americans. The British did not win, and historians give the credit to Galvez and to George Rogers Clark, whose well-earned luster and fame no one should attempt to dim. But it is just possible that even they, if they could, would be willing to share their pedestal with the plasmodium of malaria.

THE VOYAGE OF THE HANKEY

On the nineteenth of February, 1793, a ship called the *Hankey* arrived at the Port of St. George in the island of Grenada, one of the southernmost of the British West Indies. One must search long and hard in the medical or historical literature of the last one hundred and eighty years to find any mention of this vessel or of its epic trip. If the search is successful, the chances are overwhelming that the whole matter will be dismissed with a phrase. Surely this is unwarranted oblivion. After the Discovery itself, this westward crossing of the South Atlantic by the *Hankey* was perhaps the most fateful voyage in the history of the New World.

A formidable defense of such a statement is obviously in order. To support this contention, it is first necessary to sketch the background of the *Hankey*, and then to describe the impact of its untimely arrival in the Caribbean.

During the 1780s the anti-slavery movement in England was gaining momentum. To implement the desire on the part of many individuals to re-establish in Africa some of the freed or escaped slaves then in England or in English territories, a parcel of land was acquired in Sierra Leone. The location seemed portentous, because it was here that Sir John Hawkins had started the whole business of trading in human lives, as far as Britain was concerned, well over two hundred years before. In order to organize the project, the Sierra Leone Company was formed with many of the leading philanthropists of England at its head. Like many such enterprises, it was far more starry-eyed than practical.

When the English colonists appeared on the African coast to establish this utopia for former slaves, the reception that greeted them was not as cordial as had been anticipated. A native chief, motivated less by an urge to welcome African expatriates back to the jungle than by a desire to even some old scores with the British, burned the original town. When a later expedition was organized, it was decided to build a colony on the island of Boullam (or

Bulam) about 250 miles up the coast. The colonists, all in the best of health, embarked from England in April, 1792, on board two vessels, the *Calypso* and the *Hankey*. Contemporary accounts intimate that a profit motive as well as a crusade for reintegration stimulated these eager adventurers, and these were not the only unkind thoughts about the enterprise. In sharp contrast to everything else about the island of Boullam, the natives were distinctly cool, and the settlers, many of whom were women and children, found that the only place where they were safe was offshore on board the two ships.

For nine months, during both broiling heat and the swelters of the rainy season, the colonists stayed afloat, and many of them sickened and succumbed. On one occasion the captain took a ship to Bissao, a Portuguese settlement a short distance away, to get some decent water. During that brief trip, nine of the crew of twelve became suddenly feverish and died. The mortality continued, and finally it became apparent that to remain was hopeless. Of the more than two hundred persons who had left England, scarcely one-fourth of them were still alive; so the survivors, with no more than a skeleton crew, put out to sea in the *Hankey*. Because of the condition of the ship and the sailors, it was unthinkable to set out for home; but after great difficulty they succeeded in getting to the Cape Verde Islands. Two British warships were anchored there, and the captain of one took pity on his sorry countrymen. He sent men on board to repair the tattered rigging and then loaned the distressed ship four seamen to help it on its way. Seldom has kindness been so poorly rewarded. Two of these sailors died before the wretched vessel had been at sea more than a few days, while back on the warships forty-five crew men grew feverish, turned yellow, vomited black blood and perished. In the meantime the *Hankey* sailed on, carrying to Grenada its cargo of yellow fever.

Cases soon began to appear along the waterfront in St. George, and from the beginning of March until the end of

May, two hundred sailors manning ships in the trade between Grenada and the rest of the world died of the fever.
In addition, there were those on board the "Guinea ships,"
the slavers, anchored in the bay who also contracted the
disease and failed to recover. By the middle of April the
epidemic was established onshore. Note was made of the
distressing fact that camphor, sewed into a small linen bag
and hung around the neck, offered no protection. While
the epidemic raged, two out of every three of the white
civilian inhabitants became ill and fully twenty percent of
these died. The infection also spread to the military garrison on the island and created havoc there.

The island was thoroughly infested with the sickness;
and a contemporary account makes the following significant statement, "But the infection was not confined to
Grenada alone; from this, as a focus, it spread to the other
islands, to Jamaica, St. Domingo, and Philadelphia by
means of vessels on board of which the infection was
retained. . . ." The yellow fever epidemic of 1793 in Philadelphia has been described many times. That is another
story and does not concern us now. We are particularly
interested in the remark, "it spread to the other islands, to
Jamaica, St. Domingo. . . ."

It may seem, at this point, that the voyage of the
Hankey is suffering from overemphasis. Time and time
again epidemic disease has been introduced into strange
lands and has swept away susceptible people. There is
tragedy in plenty, but nothing very remarkable about such
an event. Even less startling is the knowledge that yellow
fever had been present in the Caribbean several times
before. There are two important facts, however, that must
be recognized. First, yellow fever, in its own characteristic
fashion, had disappeared from most of the Caribbean area
quite some years prior to 1793. Second, and this is the
crucial point, the timing of its reintroduction was most
fortuitous, and decisive.

The *Aedes* mosquito is an excellent sailor, and it had a
peculiar fondness for wooden ships. It would breed in the

buckets and in the bilge, and it would bite wherever human blood could be found. So, as a biologic agent, the *Hankey* carried the recently infected individuals and the mosquitoes to a suitable climate where there was a sizeable population of susceptible individuals. But most important of all, a continuing supply of nonimmunes was guaranteed by the fact that this particular time marked the beginning of a decade of almost uninterrupted military activity in the Caribbean.

In the War of the French Revolution, Pitt determined to strike at the economic resources of France by picking up her colonies in the West Indies. One of the early British actions consisted of sending seven hundred men from Jamaica to St. Domingo where St. Nicholas Mole was taken without a fight. Several small towns nearby surrendered, but the troops began to get sick and the commander had difficulty finding men to garrison the new acquisitions. Because of the high morbidity and relatively low mortality, the evidence suggests that at this time, malaria was the villain.

The following year the inhabitants revolted against the English and the situation became grave. In May, 1794, sixteen hundred men under Major General Whyte arrived, and early in June Port-au-Prince, the capital of French St. Domingo, was captured. More troops soon arrived; but although about 460 had been sent from Guadeloupe where yellow fever was now rampant, more than a hundred had been thrown into the sea on the way and another one hundred fifty had been landed at Jamaica to die. The rest of the force began to sicken equally fast. On the 29th of June the seven battalions in St. Domingo had more than 1,700 men on the sick list and only 2,000 in health. By the seventeenth of July, thirty-four out of sixty-four of the recently landed officers were dead. Yellow fever had now taken charge of the campaign, and by the end of July all military operations were necessarily suspended. The havoc continued through the autumn and by New Year's, 1795, the seven battalions in the island had dwindled to about eighteen hundred of all ranks, and of these less than eleven hundred were fit for duty.

Many more troops had been sent out from England who were intended eventually for St. Domingo. They never arrived and the reason is simply that the same fate caught up with them elsewhere. Late in 1793 General Grey had been ordered to foreign service with a force of seven thousand men. He was to attack Martinique, Guadeloupe, and St. Lucia and then proceed to St. Domingo. He took the three islands in the spring of 1794, but in a few months his army was decimated. Of the officers who sailed with Grey to Martinique, twenty-seven were killed or died of their wounds, and 170 died of tropical disease, especially yellow fever. Five thousand of his original seven thousand troops went to their graves for the same cause.

Reinforcements were procured, however, and by June 1, 1795, there were three thousand British soldiers on the island; but seventeen hundred of them were too ill to be under arms. In spite of the fact that more men were poured into the pest-ridden place in the next two months, by the end of that time there were only two thousand living troops, half of whom were sick. On shipboard the mortality was even worse than onshore. At one time, when British battleships were actually anchored at the Mole, two French frigates made a daring raid only a short distance from the port and captured an ordnance ship and five transports with four hundred troops on board. His Majesty's proud and powerful fleet was utterly paralyzed by mosquitoes.

The dreary story drags on until finally General Maitland, facing on his own responsibility the realization that conditions were completely hopeless, entered into an agreement with Toussaint L'Ouverture and evacuated St. Domingo in October, 1798.

For the United States the significance of this debacle lies in the fact that the Louisiana Territory, now in the somewhat tremulous grasp of Spain, was again a definite objective of Britain. Earlier, as we have seen, there had been English attempts to colonize along the Mississippi. During this era there were multiple intrigues, including a prospective attack on the lower Mississippi Valley sponsored by the British, but manned by American frontiersmen. With England at war with Spain the conclusion is inescapable that if British manpower had not been swallowed up in futile warfare in the pestilent West Indies, Louisiana would again have become a military objective and probably would have fallen to England. Fortescue, the eminent British military historian, says, "The secret of England's impotence for the first six years of the war may be said to lie in the two fatal words, St. Domingo."

After this the French returned to center stage in St. Domingo. While the previous events had been going on, Spain had ceded to France her part of the island. There have been in recorded history more valuable gifts, for by now Toussaint L'Ouverture was in full control of the island. He recognized the right of the Directory to keep a civil agent—the citizen Roume—as a check on his power, but actually Roume was helplessly in L'Ouverture's power. As soon as Rigaud, his mulatto rival, was crushed, Toussaint imprisoned Roume and soon thereafter seized by force the Spanish part of the island. He now gave a new constitution to St. Domingo, as Napoleon had done to France after the 18th Brumaire, by which he not only assumed all political power for life, but he also ascribed to himself the right to name his own successor. By his own denomination, he was, "First of the Blacks" and the Bonaparte of the Antilles. His actions were dramatic, and in many respects admirable, but they were hardly prudent. To Napoleon, this behavior was sheer mockery.

The First Consul, however, had other reasons than mere vengeance for liquidating the power of Toussaint. Napoleon needed St. Domingo as the one place from which he could rebuild the colonial system of France. Furthermore, and he realized it full well, he needed St. Domingo in order to reach and hold Louisiana. Toussaint would have to be crushed.

Napoleon detailed to the mission twenty thousand of his best troops, men who had fought under him in the Alps and in Italy. Leclerc, who had married Napoleon's sister Pauline, had the command. The general was advised by his medical officers to garrison his troops at Plaisance and other towns at high altitudes where yellow fever did not exist; but Napoleon had given his brother-in-law a tight timetable to follow, one which would not allow a leisurely campaign from mountain strongholds. He was to carry out his mission in three periods. First, he must occupy the coast towns and ready his columns there in fifteen to twenty days. The second movement would be one of rapid, converging blows from several points to shatter organized resistance. Then mobile flying columns must rout the fugitive black bands out of the forests and the mountains.

Leclerc arrived off Cape Samana in Spanish Hispaniola on January 29, 1802, with twelve thousand of his splendidly equipped force. He split the expedition into four groups that attained their objectives within a week. The second division arrived from France and on February 17 the interior was invaded by four different attacking forces. By March 24 the last stronghold of the blacks had been captured, and by early May, Christophe, Dessalines, and Toussaint had all capitulated.

Leclerc had lost five thousand men in his brief but sanguinary campaign. Furthermore, there were five thousand others in hospital suffering from wounds, malaria and enteric diseases. But that was unimportant. What was important was that the finest army of Europe had demonstrated in St. Domingo its military superiority over a mob of former slaves.

In May the rains came, and as the mists rose from the towns and villages and bivouacs, from every broken calabash and from every cistern and trough, the avengers of the blacks took wing. All that summer long the yellow fever lashed the conquerors of St. Domingo. French troops and sailors of the fleet were stricken by the hundreds each day. In a month three thousand were dead, and this ruinous quota increased as the months wore on. The army, already weakened by casualties, was paralyzed, and the reinforcements from France helped not a whit. The late-comers—Poles, Germans and Netherlanders, for the most part—immediately contracted the fever and died faster than the French. Leclerc, at this point, became dependent on the dubious loyalty of his black troops. In June, Toussaint was taken by a ruse and sent to France to die in a miserable prison. Then the news leaked out that slavery had been re-established in Guadeloupe, and the black revolution flared again. Leclerc, suffering from the fevers of malaria and the flirtations of Pauline, sent home reports begging for more money and more troops. By this time the rebel generals began to see the situation in a new light. The mortality from yellow fever had soared to an appalling figure. The time appeared ripe to take advantage of it. One regiment that had landed from Europe 1,395 strong had only 190 men left alive, and of these, 107 were in hospital. Another regiment had landed 1,000 strong and now numbered 150 of whom 133 were in hospital. With such military impotence obvious to them on every hand, the black chiefs, led by Dessalines and Christophe, deserted Leclerc and resumed their leadership of the masses.

By the middle of November the French were in desperate straits. They held about a half dozen important coast towns; the interior had been lost to the blacks; forty thousand soldiers, sailors and civilians had been buried; and Leclerc himself was dead of yellow fever.

Back in June when the reports of the early successes had reached Napoleon and fortune seemed to be smiling broadly on his enterprises, he had ostensibly ordered an expedition to prepare for the reinforcement of Leclerc; actually, it was destined for New Orleans. If these projects had succeeded, France would have held a great colonial empire in North America protected by the naval and military base of St. Domingo. All through the fall these plans went forward. General Victor was gathering men, ships and supplies in Holland for the venture. Before he could sail, however, he was icebound.

In the first week of January, 1803, Napoleon received the news of Leclerc's death and the forlorn state to which his proud legions in St. Domingo had fallen. Napoleon did not take long to change his mind. "It was known," according to Barbe-Marbois, "on the 20th of February 1803, and before Mr. Monroe had sailed for Europe, that the commander of the squadron on board of which the division of troops intended for Louisiana was embarked, had received orders to postpone his departure."

On April 11 Napoleon was telling Talleyrand, "Irresolution and deliberation are no longer in season. I renounce Louisiana. It is not only New Orleans that I cede: it is the whole colony, without reserve; I know the price of what I abandon . . . I direct you to negotiate the affair."

So the Louisiana Territory became a part of the United States, and it is well recognized that this was of overwhelming importance to the future of the floundering republic that would one day become the most powerful nation on earth. The role of yellow fever in this drama has never been appreciated, but it was decisive. Considering the ultimate results on the subsequent history of three great nations, it is fascinating to reflect on the part played by the unheralded and unsung voyage of the fever-ridden, forgotten little *Hankey* which, so many years ago, carried a cargo of destiny to a distant and little known port.

7

A Tinge of Sallowness

In the decades between 1820 and 1860 the republic might be said to have advanced from a teenage innocence into an adult maturity, and one ripening factor that should not be overlooked was infectious disease. The important ailments then of most concern were not, for the most part, the "usual childhood diseases" that commonly afflict the growing individual at the present time. Many of the great scourges of that day the majority of modern physicians have never encountered outside a textbook. As disease entities they outdid themselves for by their very viciousness and their proclivity for terror they brought about their own extermination.

The great political and economic issues facing the nation in the period under discussion were such matters as growth and expansion, the abolition of slavery, and laying the foundation for a western empire. It was also a time when the minds of ordinary men began to stretch, when ideas became tools rather than ivory tower musings, when education was no longer only the prerogative of the upper class, when mechanical inventiveness burgeoned, when the realization dawned on the multitude that fate was not foreordained, and most important of all, that something could actually be done about controlling the ravages of epidemic disease.

It is true that it would take a lot of doing and the cost would be great in effort and in life, but until these concepts were understood, nothing of moment could be done. It is quite possible that disease had its most far-reaching and decisive influence on ideas during these decades. Without question there was ample opportunity for such inducement to be brought to bear. The era we are about to consider was the sickliest in the entire history of the United States.

It makes little difference what part of the nation is contemplated. The rugged pioneer and his sturdy wife comprise a fiction for which the artist and the sculptor have a genuine fondness. In reality all this amounts to no more than a parable and has no foundation whatsoever in medical or historic fact. The traditionally tough, axe-swinging frontiersman and his equally hardy helpmate are part of the mythology of our pioneer life. As it turned out, the brave pioneers spent much of their time burying one another, or lying on their own sickbeds beset by malaria, typhoid fever, diphtheria, erysipelas, tuberculosis, milk-sickness, pneumonia, yellow fever, smallpox and cholera, to name but a few common afflictions. They lived in squalor, drank dirty water, ate infected food; their cattle were diseased, their clothing was inadequate, their housing was abominable and their lives were miserable and marginal.

It should not be assumed, however, that only the poor were victims. The English novelist, Frederick Marryat, paid a visit to this country in the years 1837–38. In *A Diary In America,* published after his return home, he gives a vivid picture of his experiences. "It must be understood that during the unhealthy season in the southern states on the Mississippi, the planters, cotton-growers, slave-holders, store-keepers, and indeed almost every class, excepting the slaves and overseers, migrate to the northward, to escape the yellow fever and spend a portion of their gains in amusement." He further states:

> I may here remark that the two states, Illinois and Indiana, and the western portions of Kentucky and Tennessee are very unhealthy; not a year passes without a great mortality from the

bilious congestive fever, a variety of the yellow fever, and the
ague—more especially Illinois and Indiana, with the western
portion of Ohio, which is equally flat with the other two
states. . . . Many and many thousands of poor Irish emigrants,
and settlers also, have been struck down by disease, never to rise
again, in these rich but unhealthy states, to which, stimulated by
the works published by land-speculators, thousands and thousands every year repair and, notwithstanding the annual expen-
diture of life, rapidly increase the population.

Marryat's experiences were by no means unique.
Although the land advertisements and the euphoric frontier newspapers always depicted the climate as healthful
and invigorating, the gravediggers' shovels played a more
somber lament. Time after time, Michigan was described
as little more than a huge malarial swamp, and the "sod-
house" territory of Kansas, Nebraska, and the Dakotas was
swept again and again by typhoid, malaria, cholera,
pneumonia, pleurisy, smallpox, and diphtheria. Malaria
was so common that it was considered a part of life.

The outstanding physician and the most eminent
teacher of medicine in the heartland of America in the first
half of the nineteenth century was Dr. Daniel Drake. In his
era, in order to be outstanding one had to be a controversial
figure. Dr. Drake served in professorial capacities between
1817 and 1852 in Lexington, Kentucky; Cincinnati, Lexington, Philadelphia, Cincinnati; Louisville, Kentucky;
Cincinnati, Louisville, and Cincinnati. The fact that he
played a game of medical chairs in an academically belligerent age does not imply that he was merely contentious.
His inquiring mind aroused an entire generation of doctors, and his writings extended his sphere of influence far
beyond the reach of his voice. His monumental effort was
the two-volume work with the overwhelmingly ponderous
title: *A Systematic Treatise, Historical, Etiological, And
Practical, On The Principal Diseases Of The Interior Valley Of North America, As They Appear In The Caucasian,
African, Indian, and Esquimaux Varieties Of Its Population.* Needless to say, when any present-day bibliophile

has occasion to refer to the book, it is called *The Principal Diseases of the Interior Valley*. In the second volume of this work appear the following perspicuous comments, "Over most of the Interior Valley, a ruddy complexion is rare, and often replaced by a slight turbid hue, or a tinge of sallowness. When standing before the medical classes of Lexington, Louisville, and Cincinnati, composed chiefly of young men between twenty and thirty years of age, I have seen very few with plump and rosy cheeks."

If the pioneers were in bad case, their city contemporaries in many instances were even worse off. The new arrivals migrating to these shores in great numbers after the close of the Napoleonic Wars landed half dead, from Europe or the British Isles, from crowded, rat-infested transports, many members of the family having perished aboard ship. It was considered normal to have a ten percent mortality on the crossing, and frequently it was far worse.

On arrival there was no one to meet them. As a matter of fact, often when the ship sailed westward, the passengers were not even certain what their New World destination might be. Unscrupulous captains, thieving crews, dishonest agents exploited the migrants in such a fashion as to create one of the most inhuman scandals of the nineteenth century. Then in the Atlantic seaports they were jammed into teeming slums where their babies were born to die in a matter of days, where their own lives were brief, where epidemics raged, where public water supplies and municipal sewerage were political infamies, where sanitation was as yet unimagined and where literally nobody gave a damn.

During the earliest years of the nineteenth century, New York appears to have been a clean and tidy town, terms in which it has never since been described even by those most enamoured of that community. The death rate was about 25 per thousand, and the infant mortality stayed within a range of 120 to 140 per thousand live births, which in those days were favorable statistics. By the century's second quarter, man had marked the earth with ruin. The flood of immigration, the increasing number of rapidly constructed and feverishly manned factories, and the consequent surrounding slums were to typify the new era, and death strode from door to door.

A comparable situation evolved in Boston, where in the decade from 1810 to 1820 the average age of all who died in that city was 27.85 years. If that statistic seems ghastly, even taking into account the customary high mortality among infants and children, the real shocker is yet to come. During the years from 1840 to 1845 the average age at death in Boston was only 21.43 years. Equally staggering figures applied as well to New York and Philadelphia and in all instances were far worse than those of any of the cities of Europe.

The death and sickness rates in the United States were so high during the period because too many people emigrated in too short a time. It must be realized that this was not merely due to a labor vacuum in America but also because of a rapid increase in the population of Europe.

The number of inhabitants of Europe had increased only slightly from the days of Charlemagne to the beginning of the Industrial Revolution. War, famine, and pestilence had held down any telling expansion of population for a millennium, but then from an estimated 140 million people in 1750, it rose to 188 million in 1800 and to 266 million in 1850. Inasmuch as there was no particular moratorium on war and pestilence in the mid-eighteenth century, it is of some interest to explore the causes of the relatively sudden increase in the populace during this period. The explanation, according to some of our most pensive historians, was the unhonored, unsung, undramatic potato. The white potato began its prehistoric existence, as far as we are aware, in Peru. The Spaniards took it home with them soon after Pizarro had overcome the Incas. From thence the Spanish colonists took it westward again to Florida where it was soon captured by Sir John Hawkins and bundled off to Britain. The tuber, with an abundant

yield, could be grown on tiny plots of marginal land, producing several times as much in food value per acre as
could be grown in grain. In a relatively short time it had
become a popular crop in Ireland, in Lancashire, in the
Scottish Highlands and on the continent in Spain, Italy,
Germany, and the Low Countries. The areas of the most
intensive potato culture were the same areas where the
rapid increase in population was most apparent.

So in the Old World there were too many people, and
the urban and agricultural economics of Europe were
changing. The peasant, to whom a dozen acres represented virtual affluence, was being crowded off the land.
In the cities the disruptions of an industrialized society
often resulted in a maldistribution of jobs and unemploy-
ment. On the other hand, in North America there were
mills to be manned, rails to be laid, services to be rendered,
and land to be tilled. From across the Atlantic came the
immigrants by the millions, but for the most part they
traded misery for abject misery. The conditions under
which the lower classes—the vast majority of the people in
both urban and rural Europe—existed can never have
been as bad as in the early nineteenth century. They were
overworked, underfed, badly housed, and sickly. They
abandoned British and continental communities where
human degradation was indescribable to encounter circumstances, if they survived the passage, that were far
worse. Ordinarily those who came from cities tended to
stay in the cities, whereas those who had previously tilled
the soil preferred to go out on the land, but their fates were
not dissimilar.

The stage then was set for a health condition unlike
any that had ever existed on this continent. The decades
we are considering would be known as "the period of the
great epidemics." The great epidemics were of three
varieties—yellow fever, smallpox, and cholera. Influenza is
not included, not because it did not occur during these
years (on the contrary there were frequent outbreaks) but
even one in 1847 classified as a pandemic did not carry a

significant mortality rate. The influenza viruses are gregarious organisms and enjoy mingling with people, but it is only when those viruses team up alongside virulent bacteria with their own affinity for the respiratory tract that the partnership produces a highly fatal pandemic.

The first disease we will consider from this omnipotent triumvirate of afflictions is yellow fever. Because its mode of transmission was via mosquitoes, yellow fever was confined to the port cities and the nearby river valleys. In 1822, for example, there were severe epidemics of yellow fever in New York and in Pensacola. In 1824 there were 236 deaths from yellow fever in Charleston, South Carolina. During the nineteenth century, thirteen outbreaks of yellow fever were recorded in Virginia alone. The problems were bound to be the greatest in New Orleans of all the port cities. Here, the frequent invasions of yellow fever invariably stormed up the Mississippi Valley spreading death and terror along the lowlands. For close to a century, the death rate in New Orleans was far higher than the birth rate. The only way the city could maintain and increase its population was by immigration, and because of the wealth of natural resources in the region, the people continued to come despite the hazards. They came to do or die. Sometimes they did; oftener they died.

During this era, the most awesome epidemic on the Atlantic seaboard occurred in Virginia in 1855 at Portsmouth. On June 6 of that year the *Ben Franklin,* in distress from need of repairs, arrived from St. Thomas where yellow fever had been rampant when the ship had left that port. For about a month, during which the repairs to the vessel proceeded apace, nothing untoward occurred. Then suddenly a boiler worker on the ship became ill and three days later was dead of yellow fever. Soon other workers on the *Ben Franklin* sickened and died and the contagion began spreading in Plymouth. In a short time it had crossed the bay to Norfolk.

The ravages of the disease exceeded anything experienced in the Old Dominion since the early days of Jamestown. At the beginning of the epidemic, Norfolk had a population of 16,000. Six thousand persons promptly fled the city. Practically the entire remaining ten thousand, except those who had had a previous attack, suffered from the scourge. There were about two thousand deaths, and for weeks Norfolk was little more than a ghost town. Stores and business places were closed; abandoned dwellings stood bleak and deserted. The only traffic in the streets were the carriages of physicians, nurses, or the relief associations; the "sick wagons" creaked off toward the temporary hospitals, and the hearses rumbled away toward the permanent cemeteries. Surrounding towns cut themselves off from communication with the beleaguered city. The great wharves and warehouses were silent, and the only vessel afloat in the harbor was a little steamer that met the boats from Baltimore and Richmond in Hampton Roads— to bring in empty coffins.

The epidemic reached its height near the end of August and continued to wage furiously until well into September but did not end until a merciful frost on October 26. This was only the worst of several devastating epidemics of yellow fever in the South during this period.

When old Dr. Benjamin Waterhouse died in Cambridge in 1846 at the age of ninety-two, his final entry in his diary was, "I cut the claws and wings of smallpox." Some of his Massachusetts contemporaries maintained, apparently with considerable justice, that he had tried to turn in the claws to collect his bounty. In his half-page obituary in the *Boston Medical and Surgical Journal* for October 7, 1846, his contributions to "the introduction of the practice of vaccination into this country" received equal billing with his stand on tobacco. "A lecture which he delivered about 1805 to the undergraduates [Harvard, of course] on the custom of smoking cigars, is supposed to have had great influence in whatever diminution of that practice was consequent on its publication." There is something about the tone of this literary leave-taking that intimates that Dr. Waterhouse was not adored by his Bos-

ton contemporaries in quite the degree that latter-day wor-
shippers would prefer to have us believe.

Early in 1799 a copy of Edward Jenner's *An Inquiry
into the Causes and Effects of the Variolae Vaccinae* had
been sent to Waterhouse by his London friend Dr. John C.
Lettsom. The American recognized the importance of the
investigations detailed in this work and shortly wrote an
article of his own about the new inoculation method that
was published in a Boston newspaper, the *Columbian Cen-
tinel*. Waterhouse next obtained some cowpox vaccine
from another English friend, Dr. John Haygarth, and he
was in business. He tried to monopolize the trade by
licensing physicians in outlying communities to adminis-
ter material that he supplied for a sizeable cut in the take.
The metropolitan clientele Waterhouse decided to handle
himself. Unfortunately, there were flies in old Ben's un-
guent. There were other American doctors, and right in
the neighborhood, too, who had friends in Britain, and
from whom vaccine could be obtained. When this became
apparent, Waterhouse, realizing the jig was up, began to
behave more like the hero his modern acolytes delight to
depict.

Although Waterhouse was instrumental in introduc-
ing the "kine pox" into this country, the sad facts of the
matter were that the variola virus could get along very
nicely without claws or wings. At that time, the only
known method of propagating the vaccine, once it had
been derived from Old Bossy, was from one human arm to
another. This in itself could lead to complications, since
sometimes, along with immunity to smallpox, the recipient
acquired syphilis, or erysipelas, or some other virulent
dividend. The result was that in Waterhouse's era, despite
the fact that control measures were available and understood, smallpox would appear again and again, killing and
crippling as it had done for centuries. It was not until 1870,
when the first faint glimmerings of bacteriology appeared
and the first calf lymph vaccine became available, that the

hazards of extraneous infections were also eliminated and the genuine control of smallpox became feasible.

In modern America the term Asiatic cholera is only encountered by certain travelers who discover to their annoyance that in order to enter some countries they must be vaccinated against the disease. Even then its only significance is the nuisance of two subcutaneous injections and a mark on the immunization record. It was not always thus. In the nineteenth century the very words struck terror into the hearts of millions of people across the entire world. As an epidemic scourge, it has a fascinating and mystifying history.

It is commonly stated that Asiatic cholera had smouldered in endemic form in India for centuries, but Hirsch, the great German student of geographical and historical pathology, was not convinced that any outbreak prior to the devastating epidemic near Pondicherry in 1768–69 warranted that diagnosis. In any event, it was an entirely unknown threat outside the Far East prior to the nineteenth century. Whatever the motivation of the organism may have been, it apparently set out on a campaign of world conquest in 1816. In that year in the district of Behar, near Purneah, Asiatic cholera became epidemic, but it was not until August of the following year that the authorities were aware of the seriousness of the situation by which time it had spread to Calcutta and Jessore. By October the pestilence had already overrun a great part of Lower Bengal. From then on, with only occasional hesitations, the epidemic was on the march. By 1822 it had appeared in Ceylon and in Singapore, on the Zanzibar coast, the Philippines, the Chinese Empire and in Japan. Its westward march began in 1821 and two years later had extended to Syria and Persia.

Then, for some inexplicable reason, the invasion stopped. The plague appears to have died out even in Central Asia itself, and for a period of some four years the disease was again confined solely to India. The interval, however, appears to have been used for the realignment and re-grouping of the forces. The blitzkrieg was being readied. The pestilence charged across the border into Persia for the second time in 1829. Shortly it was in Teheran, which previously had escaped, and well before the end of 1830 the contagion was well established on the soil of Russia, and by June of 1831 had attacked St. Petersburg. By the same year, also, it was in Germany and from there it was a short hop to Britain. By December it had appeared in Scotland and shortly thereafter it was firmly established in Belfast, Dublin, and Cork.

Needless to say, this inexorable advance had been watched with trepidation in America. In Canada the impe-rial authorities had taken steps to try to prevent the inva-sion of the disease. At the time, an enormous influx of people from England and Ireland was entering Canada. Grosse Isle, twenty-seven miles east of Quebec in the St. Lawrence and directly astride the path of incoming steam-ers from Europe, was chosen for the purpose of quaran-tine, and "a battery of two twelve, and one eighteen, pound guns in the centre of the island facing the river" despite its formidable appearance, somehow failed to halt the cholera vibrio in its passage upstream to Quebec. In that year of 1832 "fifty one thousand seven hundred immigrants from England and Ireland arrived at the port of Quebec, and in every city whence these immigrants came cholera was epidemic." On April 28, 1832, the ship *Constantia* from Limerick arrived at Grosse Isle with 170 immigrants aboard, 29 deaths from cholera having occurred during the voyage. Within the next few weeks a number of other vessels with a cargo of cholera disembarked their infected passengers on the island, but by June 8 the disease was in Quebec, and a day later in Montreal.

Within a week cholera had appeared in Whitehall, New York, and it presented itself in Mechanicsville and Ogdensburg in a matter of days. The first case of cholera in New York City was not recorded until the end of June, but in those days the Board of Health had acquired no fame for its courageous and forthright approach to minor issues, to say nothing of major crises. There is good reason to believe that the disease had been imported there at least as soon as it had arrived in Canada, but the Board of Health, for reasons of its own, declined to present any extravagant claim for priority.

In the meantime there was a war on in the United States. As such things go it was a very weird war. It was named for an Indian leader called Black Hawk, who had courage and leadership (but possibly not very much sense) and doubtless a righteous cause because the old problem of land rights was again paramount. Furthermore, it was the last of the Indian conflicts that would occur in the Old Northwest, and hence it would be an object of unbounded affection in the territory involved. Finally it was the outstanding example of the one-act play with the all-star cast. Included in the dramatis personae would be characters later to assume stellar roles, such as Abraham Lincoln, Zachary Taylor, Jefferson Davis, Winfield Scott, Albert Sidney Johnston, and Joseph E. Johnston as well as several who would never quite become headliners, including General John Reynolds, who, a generation later, would fall leading his command on the first day at Gettysburg.

Still, there was a war on, and during the latter part of June, 1832, various detachments of regulars were sent from the Atlantic coast to Chicago. At Buffalo four steamers were available for the embarkation of the troops. Suddenly while the vessels were passing up the Great Lakes, Asiatic cholera appeared among the soldiers. This was a far more potent enemy than the hostile Indian could ever have been. The expedition was totally disrupted. Two of the vessels got no farther than Fort Gratiot, where the utter virulence of the pestilence compelled the soldiers to land. The ravages among the men of the detachment of Colonel Twiggs, who landed at this spot, were so ghastly as to banish military discipline to the winds. Those of the command who were able to assemble simply dispersed in every direction. They ran for the byways and they ran for the woods. Terrified inhabitants of the area refused them shelter or food or comfort. They carried contagion; they were burdened with death. And so along the rutted roadways, beside the turbulent streams and in the woods and in the fields, they died. No one comforted their last moments because no one was there. No one marked their graves because no one buried them. No one concerned themselves about medals, or pensions, or honors because these men had run away. The fact that they had run from something more terrifying than enemy fire, more mystifying than military combat was beside the point. They were to be shunned at any cost.

It so happened that no fatalities occurred on board the *Sheldon Thompson,* the steamer on which General Scott had embarked, until Mackinac had been passed and Lake Michigan entered. Before leaving New York, Scott had become sufficiently concerned about the possibility of this new plague striking his men that he had learned as much about it as he could from the army surgeon stationed there. When the disease did appear, it was with sudden and fatal violence. Crew and cargo became jittery, as well as the only surgeon on board. The latter took to his bed with a bottle of wine, leaving Scott to apply his newly acquired clinical knowledge. This he did with sufficient aplomb so that a general panic was averted.

Although cholera was present in Chicago, it stopped spreading by the end of July. Before any significant contingent of Scott's force could be brought into action, the conflict had been finished by the Illinois militia and some regulars at Bad Axe.

Back in New York, the month of July was grim indeed. The Medical Society, furious at the dilatory Board of Health, announced on July 2 that there had already been nine cases of cholera with only one survival. The death toll mounted rapidly and panic spread. On the tenth there were forty-five deaths. Business stagnated and more than 70,000 people, about a third of the population, fled the city.

During that summer, there were 3,500 deaths from cholera in New York.

In Philadelphia the situation was far better. One reason was that much of the city was supplied with good water pumped in by steam engines through pipelines from the Schuylkill River at Fairmont, and the streets and alleyways were kept clean by using an ample amount of water. Even so there were nine hundred deaths, most of them in the slums and the poor sections and in the Arch Street prison, which became a shambles.

There were 853 deaths from cholera in Baltimore and 831 in Cincinnati, but of all the places in the world for a waterborne epidemic to thrive, none was so ideally situated as New Orleans, and the vibrio took full advantage of the terrain. The highest ground was that along the levee so that the river was higher than the elevation of the city, which, in turn, was higher than Lake Ponchartrain. Periodically the gutters in the city streets were flushed with river water. This was accomplished by opening gates into tunnels through the levee, allowing the water to wash the filth of the streets out into the swamps and bayous toward the lake. The ground water level was literally just below the surface of the land, and wells, both public and private, supplied water for the city. Add to this picture the ubiquitous backhouse and it would be difficult to conceive a simpler and more effective manner in which the water supply of an entire community could be contaminated.

Cholera approached New Orleans in a leisurely fashion, and unlike yellow fever, it did not arrive from the Gulf but rather came down the Ohio and then the Mississippi. It arrived on the twenty-fifth of October and liked what it saw. Two days later it was in every part of the city. During the previous summer there had been a considerable exodus because of yellow fever, but now the flight from the pest-ridden area was headlong so that scarcely 35,000 persons remained from a population of at least 50,000. In little more than two weeks 6,000 were dead, a

frightful mortality of one in every six of those who would
not or could not abandon their homes.

The holocaust was soon over, but the infection smouldered all winter and was spread by waterborne traffic to
the towns on the Gulf coast as well as to the West Indies.
There was a sudden flare-up again in the spring, and it
required only three weeks to take another thousand lives.
In addition, there were many deaths in the towns and on
the plantations of the lower parishes and a terrific loss of
life among the slaves.

The second great invasion of cholera occurred in 1849.
As in the first, the starting focus was India, where at
Calcutta a particularly virulent strain of the disease had
made its appearance in 1840, and thence passed through
China to Siberia and on to Russia, where during 1847–48
more than a million persons succumbed. From the Near
East the epidemic spread to the Mediterranean areas. In
France 150,000 died. Cholera soon appeared in Germany,
and it was from this area that most emigration to America
was coming at that time.

Several groups of Germans, some of whom were from
infected areas, appeared at the port of Le Havre in the
autumn of 1848, seeking transportation to the New World.
Two hundred and eighty steerage passengers aboard the
Swanton left the French port on October 31, 1848, bound
for New Orleans. After twenty-seven days at sea, there was
an outbreak of cholera on board, and when the ship arrived
at New Orleans on December 11, there had been sixteen
deaths among the passengers. Again the city was ravaged
by the pestilence, but this time it was carried by the river
boats up the Mississippi, scattering riparian carnage, and
up the Ohio to Cincinnati, where in a city of 110,000, there
were nearly 6,000 deaths.

But this time there would be still another difference,
for this time the pestilence would be spread even more by
land than by water. This was the year of the Forty-niners,
and for every lusty adventurer who set forth seeking the
elusive pot of gold who died of exposure, or injury or

Indian assault, a thousand would leave their whitening bones along the western trails, struck down by cholera.

During 1849–50, cholera seems to have affected every group or company that traveled the Oregon Trail. Major Osborne Cross, bound for Oregon, wrote on May 26, 1849, that in many instances nearly entire parties of emigrants had succumbed to the ravages of this disease. Another pioneer, George H. Himes, estimated that prior to 1849, 30,000 Oregon immigrants had died of cholera west of the Missouri River. Himes also reported that in 1853 he saw the remains of a train of fifteen or twenty wagons on the Platte River whose members were said to have died of "plains cholera."

A diary of 1852 states, "All along the road up the Platte River was a graveyard; almost any time of day you could see people burying their dead; some places five or six graves in a row, with board head signs. . . ." On the plains the illness usually lasted only one day. Those who arose in the morning feeling well died before nightfall. Wagons, beds, blankets, and household goods were abandoned by the side of the trail. They had no value, they had no interest for any human being. Not even the Indians dared to touch them.

Cholera struck severely in California and was documented by the following contemporary comment dated Sacramento December 8, 1850, "We now walked over to the back part of town, and visited the burial ground where I saw the long parallel lines of graves of cholera victims. These mournful heaps of sand were the resting places of upwards of 1700 persons, who had fallen in 15 months; 900 of them in 3 weeks." However, despite the carnage along the Oregon Trail, cholera apparently did not reach Oregon. The formidable desert barrier of Wyoming, Idaho, and eastern Oregon itself was too stern for the vibrio, and actually the ramparts to the east of the gold fields of California were probably impenetrable. Cholera presumably reached California by sea.

In 1854 cholera disappeared from the United States as

abruptly, and apparently with as little reason as it had in 1834, and was not to return until 1866. On this occasion, New York, New Orleans, and St. Louis were particularly hard hit, but this was a relatively mild epidemic in contrast to the two preceding episodes. To complete the picture there was one more appearance in 1873, limited to the Mississippi River valley.

Despite the fact that Asiatic cholera has been, as an epidemic scourge, of no significance whatsoever on this continent for a century, it would be a serious mistake to ascribe to this once highly fatal disease a minor role in our total social development.

The disease was influential far beyond the horror of its mortality. It thrived primarily because of dirt, filth and poverty, and when the wealthy and the aristocratic were afflicted, it was usually because their standards of cleanliness had fallen below their affectations. Cholera traveled widely and rapidly because of an unprecedented increase in trade and transportation. Steamships were replacing sail. Large numbers of people were on the move. Cities, both in the Old World and the New, had growing pains. A city is an entirely different organism from a large village, and the cholera epidemics of the nineteenth century provided much of the required impetus eventually to overcome centuries of civic indifference and inertia regarding matters of sanitation and public health. In America, these epidemics were bound to make a profound impression. This nation was not inclined to take tyranny for granted, even if the tyranny sprang from an unrecognized and microscopic foe. Even though the exact mechanism may not have been apparent, the fact that there was an indubitable correlation between the incidence of cholera and the existence of slums, slime and sewage stimulated not only the theories upon which the public health movement was founded, but gave a forward thrust to its practical applications.

Death is a dramatic occurrence when it is sudden. Epidemics are similarly dramatic and horror-inspiring events because of the speed with which they strike and spread. But the individual is just as dead and the loss to family, friends and community is just as great if the Reaper approaches with a slower gait. It is important, therefore, to note that despite the stress placed on epidemics in these pages and despite the terror resulting from them, the principal causes of death during these decades were not cholera, smallpox, and yellow fever, but instead were ailments that were constantly harassing the nation's inhabitants. These were pulmonary tuberculosis, the diarrheal diseases of infancy, bacillary dysentery, typhoid fever, lobar pneumonia, the infectious diseases of childhood, particularly scarlet fever and diphtheria, and then, the most infectious disease of all—malaria.

At this point an interpretive word or two about our ancestors might be in order. The fact, for example, that they were quickly felled by scarlet fever does not mean that they were pushovers for the trivial infection as we know that disease commonly is today. The organism was similar, but it was then a vicious and potent *Streptococcus* frequently producing a fatal septicemia or at least crippling pulmonary, mastoid, or brain abscesses. It is entirely possible, too, that the typhoid and tubercle bacilli were lustier organisms then than they are now. Certainly some strange and unexplained things happened to the death rate from tuberculosis. For example, the mortality rate from this disease for the combined populations of Boston, New York, and Philadelphia in the year 1830 was roughly 400 per 100,000 people. However, the disease began to decline long before its cause was recognized and before any specific measures to combat its dissemination had been devised. By 1900 when the first attempts at control of the disease by public health measures were initiated, the annual mortality due to the white plague in both England and America had already fallen to 200 per 100,000 population.

The situation regarding the diarrheal diseases is more easily explained. In these modern days, when every domesticated vacuum tube and transistor exudes a miasma of soap slogans and detergent diatribes, it is difficult for us to conceive of the utter nastiness wherein our forebears dwelt. Cesspools were uncovered and slaughterhouses were unscreened. In the grocery stores, worms crawled in the corn meal and ants in the sugar barrel. Wells were polluted, milk was dirty, horse manure littered the streets, flies abounded and were ignored and babies died of diarrhea and strong men died of typhoid fever.

The wide and rapid dissemination of malaria is also easily explained. The rivers were the principal routes of travel as settlers in ever increasing numbers moved westward after the Revolution, and for that reason most of them took advantage of the opportunity of acquiring the parasite along the way. Furthermore, they tended to settle along the low-lying land adjacent to rivers, where transportation was available, the land was fertile and there was access to timber and fuel and *Anopheles* mosquitoes. For many years the upland regions and the great prairies were avoided because they were considered to be lacking in these essentials.

So now what were our nineteenth-century ancestors doing about the grim problems in pathology that were facing them? As might be expected, they were meeting the issues with diverse solutions. The reasons why are not hard to find. The physician of that day was trained to care for individuals and to treat symptoms. The concept of diseases as entities, or a philosophy for their prevention were, for the most part, ideas that were still waiting in the wings. During the eighteenth and early nineteenth centuries, an incredibly useless and often harmful therapy based on utter ignorance of fundamental etiology and absolute misconceptions about pathologic physiology produced a therapeutic schema that insisted something positive must be done; otherwise the physician would have been no more useful or respected than the housewife with her home remedies. This was the era of the bleedings, the purges, the emetics, the mercurials. Even a generation or two ago, this doctrine was echoed by one medical school professor who advised his graduates, "When you are called, go. When you get there, do something."

There were a few contemporary physicians who cringed at the therapeutic violence they observed. In 1835, the Annual Discourse, an event that is still a prominent feature of the annual meeting of the Massachusetts Medical Society, was delivered by Dr. Jacob Bigelow, the professor of materia medica at Harvard. His discussion, even now regarded as a landmark in the distinguished history of that traditional event, was entitled *On Self-Limited Diseases.* His definition follows:

> By a self-limited disease, I would be understood to express one which receives limits from its own nature, and not from foreign influences: one which, after it has obtained a foothold in the system, cannot, in the present state of our knowledge, be eradicated or abridged by art, but to which there is due a certain succession of processes, to be completed in a certain time; which time and processes may vary with the constitution and condition of the patient, and may tend to death or recovery, but are not known to be shortened or greatly changed by medical treatment.

He included chicken pox, "hooping" cough, measles, scarlet fever, smallpox and erysipelas in his list of self-limited diseases. His lecture was significant in that a respected member of the medical profession, speaking from an eminent podium, enunciated the doctrine that sometimes in medicine it was best to let sick enough alone.

There were other physicians of the day who were trying to look beyond the problem of the sick individual and who were trying to influence their colleagues to improve their handling of patients. Dr. Oliver Wendell Holmes entertained his brethren and the public all his life, but he did make one original contribution to scientific medicine in 1843 at the age of thirty-three when he read a paper entitled *On the Contagiousness of Puerperal Fever* to the Boston Society for Medical Improvement. His forthright conclusions antedated by five years the intensive study by Semmelweis in Vienna and came twenty-five years before the historic revelations by Pasteur in France.

The contributions of Bigelow and Holmes gained attention because they were equipped with a sounding board. They were professors and they were in a medical center. Daniel Drake and others also obtained publicity for their views because of their positions. There were those, however, whose concepts were equally commanding but whose influence remained entirely parochial. This was because it was just as true then as it is now: It matters not whether *something* is said, but only if *someone* says it.

Dr. John Sappington is a case in point. Dr. Sappington was not a member of any noted faculty in Boston or New York or Philadelphia or even Louisiana. He was a practitioner in Arrow Rock, Missouri, and he deserves better of posterity than mere oblivion. As a young man, originally living in Tennessee, he practiced medicine for a time following some tutelage from his father and brother, both of whom were physicians. When, sometime later, he enrolled as a medical student and spent five months at the University of Pennsylvania in 1814–15, he made it quite plain to his professors that he disagreed entirely with the teachings of the time favoring bleeding, cupping, and purging in the treatment of fevers. After all, he had had some very worthwhile experience in these matters.

Fortunately for Dr. Sappington and for his patients in the Mississippi Valley, where he was destined to settle and to practice following his brief academic exposure, he was not compelled to make a career of therapeutic nihilism. In 1820 two Parisian pharmacists named Pelletier and Caventou succeeded in extracting the alkaloid quinine from Peruvian bark. By 1823 a quinine factory had been established in Philadelphia.

For reasons that are now difficult to grasp, quinine was accepted very grudgingly by the regular medical profession. It seems especially perplexing that such an attitude should prevail when "the bark" from which the active principal was derived by the French pharmacists had long enjoyed a favorable reputation for the treatment of "the ague," especially in America.

There are two possible explanations for this diffidence among the medical practitioners of the day. The first is, quinine is of no value whatsoever in other febrile conditions. Unless the doctor was a keen observer, and very familiar with the disease, he probably did not differentiate malaria from other fever-producing disorders. In such situations, when he used the drug for other infections there was no benefit obtained. The other possibility was that he used too much of the drug. The amount of quinine in "the bark" is relatively small and requires much more material to be swallowed than in the purified extract. If that fact was not recognized, there may well have been serious symptoms of toxicity. One other note might be worth mentioning. "Fever" was diagnosed by observation. The clinical thermometer would not be invented for several years.

Dr. Sappington, it should be noted, was neither the first nor the only advoacte of the drug in this country, but, as it happened, over a large area and for a considerable length of time he was by far the most effective advocate. The reasons are easily apparent and are a tribute to his resourcefulness. When Sappington began prescribing quinine openly for his ague-ridden patients along the flatlands bordering the great river, he found he was running into implacable antagonism on the part of his professional brethren who refused to budge from their insistence on depletion—that is bleeding, purging, etc.—in the treatment of fevers.

This frontier physician's solution to this therapeutic dilemma was direct and highly profitable. He simply devised a medication of his own and sold it as Dr. Sappington's Anti-Fever Pills. Forty pills cost $1.50, and an eager staff of "drummers" went on the road in the river towns to hawk the medicinal merchandise. To remind the malaria-infected populace of the importance of taking Dr. Sappington's pills, the village bells in many of the communities along the Mississippi were rung at dusk. It would appear that the musical commercial is old stuff.

In ten years he is said to have sold over a million boxes of his remedy in the western and southern states as well as in the Republic of Texas, until he decided that he had proven his point and was ready to announce the contents of his miracle drug. When he did so he stated:

. . . . the following is the author's formula:

 R Sulphate of quinine, ... 40 grains
   Gum myrrh, ... 10   "
   Liquorice, ... 30   "

Triturate well; moisten with a little water, and add just enough of the oil of sassafras to impart an agreeable odor; Divide into forty pills . . . Dose; one pill; to be repeated every one or two hours, or longer, to suit the case.

Despite the fact that nowadays, with our complex and involved ethical and professional concern about secret remedies and huckstering procedures, the marketing methods then employed would be looked upon as utterly indefensible, nevertheless Dr. Sappington and his pills probably saved more lives and did more to forward the settlement of the lower Mississippi Valley than any other men or measures of the time.

There was another example of high level pioneer-doctor public health work of the same period in the Midwest that has been largely forgotten. This incident concerned a peculiarly regionalized ailment that was responsible for killing or disabling thousands of individuals each year, caused the abandonment of many a village and farm, and significantly retarded the settlement of large Midwestern areas.

The disease was milk-sickness, or trembles, and was known by various other names. It occurred in Ohio, Indiana, Illinois, West Virginia, Kentucky, and Tennessee and in contiguous areas of bordering states. It had been recognized as early as Revolutionary days, but it did not become an important affliction until the nineteenth century when settlement beyond the Alleghenies began in earnest.

It was a strange and puzzling malady. It was generally recognized that eating the meat or drinking the milk of affected cattle was the means of communicating the disease to man. The cows themselves were not obviously ill, which naturally obscured the source of the trouble. The disease in man was marked by abdominal pain, nausea, vomiting, fever, and intense thirst. There was restlessness, irritability and frequently coma, convulsions, and death.

A more poignant situation even than that of Dr. Sappington is the case of the woman who could have solved the milk-sickness problem all by herself, and almost did. She has no medals, she has no memorials, and she is completely forgotten. Her name was Anna Pierce.

Anna Pierce as a teenage girl was brought by her family to southeastern Illinois where at the time there were no medical practitioners. She was of an independent mind and decided to become one herself. This decision required more than ordinary mental independence because medical schools, as we have noted before, simply were not open to women. Regardless of that obstacle, Anna went to Philadelphia, studied midwifery, which was allowable, nursing, and a little dentistry and then came back to practice in Illinois. Sometime after her return she married a local farmer, Jefferson Hobbs, whose sister and Anna's mother, shortly died of milk-sickness. This was prime motivation for the young practitioner to take on this fatal affliction as a personal adversary.

Despite the sparseness of her education, Dr. Anna was a keen clinical observer. She noted that both men and animals acquiring the ailment had been drinking milk or eating butter, that the epidemic was seasonal (from June until the first frost) and that milking cows did not become ill. She was now convinced that the poison that killed calves and people spared the cows because they ridded themselves of it by way of the milk glands. But if the poison came from some plant in the pasture, why were horses, sheep, and goats not ordinarily affected? Anna Hobbs knew enough about animals to appreciate that cattle eat all sorts of vegetation, whereas horses eat only grass, and even goats and sheep, despite popular concepts to the contrary, are selective in their diet.

One autumn day, in about 1834, an old Indian medicine woman showed Dr. Anna Hobbs the white snake root plants growing in the pastures that she said were the cause of milk-sickness. Anna's husband fed the herb to a calf that promptly developed the trembles. As far as is known, Anna never wrote any learned treatise about her discovery, and if she had, probably no one would have printed it. She did, however, do something that was of more immediate effect. She rounded up the men and boys in the area and started them on a campaign of weed eradication. White snake root was uprooted and burned for miles around, and in three years the plant and the disease were virtually eliminated from southeastern Illinois.

That is the pleasant part of the story. The grim aspect is that Anna was soon forgotten, others who rediscovered the same fact were ignored, and milk-sickness continued to plague localities in the Midwest for two generations. It is now known that tremetol, a toxin occurring in white snake root and in rayless goldenrod, is the substance that causes this miserable malady. It is ironic that the gradual elimination of this disease was due to the incidental improvement of pasturage rather than to any widespread understanding of the primary etiology of the ailment. It is also ironic that in 1892, almost sixty years after Anna Hobbs had demonstrated the cause of the disease and had shown how it could be eliminated, Dr. William Osler, in his famous *Practice of Medicine*, could say, "Nothing definite is known as to the cause of the disease."

Among the many tragedies in the course of human progress, a number of truths such as those demonstrated by Dr. Sappington and Dr. Hobbs have been long neglected because what were actually facts had been discarded by contemporary learned individuals as being mere frivolous opinions. Daniel Drake believed that poison ivy was probably responsible for milk-sickness, and his prestige perhaps postponed the elucidation of the problem for several decades.

But there were new ideas, new concepts in the whole field of human illness. Some diseases might be self-limited. Some diseases might be cured, or at least controlled, by medications such as quinine. Others might be eliminated by digging up weeds in the pasture. This was the situation in 1860. In another twenty years the whole spectrum would change and an entirely new world would open up, but that must wait. In the meantime a war must be fought to the bitter end, and it would be a war greater than anything that had yet occurred on any continent, in any era, in the history of the world.

8

War Is Hell

Washington is the paradise of paradoxes—a city of magnificent distances, but of still more magnificent discrepancies. Anything may be affirmed of it, everything denied. What it seems to be it is not; and although it is getting to be what it never was, it must always remain what it now is. It might be called a city, if it were not alternately populous and uninhabited; and it would be a widespread village, if it were not a collection of hospitals for decayed or callow politicians. It is the hibernating-place of fashion, of intelligence, of vice,—a resort without the attractions of waters either mineral or salt, where there is no bathing and no springs, but drinking in abundance and gambling in any quantity. Defenceless, as regards walls, redoubts, moats, or other fortifications, it is nevertheless the Sevastopol of the Republic, against which the allied army of Contractors and Claim-Agents incessantly lay siege. It is a great, little, splendid, mean, extravagant, poverty-stricken barrack for soldiers of fortune and votaries of folly.

This is the sardonic description of the nation's capital in the January, 1861 issue of the *Atlantic Monthly*. In a few weeks a new president would be taking office, facing a nation divided against itself, but more than that the North would be unaware of its weaknesses, unsure of its strengths, uncertain of its destiny.

Democracies by their very nature are never prepared for war. They stumble into conflicts and, given the opportunity, purchase the precious commodity of time, often at great price; and, if fortune is on their side, fumble through to victory. This was doubly the situation in the spring of 1861 when two combatants came to grips, neither aware of the power or determination of the other; neither appreciating its own frailty, disorganization, or utter confusion.

194

Both sides were convinced it would be a short engagement. With the capitals of the Union and the Confederacy less than a hundred miles apart, all that would be required militarily was for the South to take Washington or the North to take Richmond. On April 15, 1861 Lincoln called for 75,000 men for service for three months. More realistically President Davis had called, and obtained, 100,000 volunteers for a year, and had summoned them early in March.

There was one old man in Washington who understood war. He was the highest ranking military officer in the country and he was seventy-five years old. His name was General Winfield Scott. He had fought his country's battles in the War of 1812, in the Black Hawk War, in various other engagements with the Indians. In the War with Mexico he had trained the young company grade officers with such names as Lee, McClellan, Grant, and Jefferson Davis who would be generals, or in one case a president, before the current conflict was ended. Old, experienced General Scott recognized that the South would be a tough adversary. For this reason he proposed a strategic outline shortly to be dubbed, and sneered at, as the Anaconda Plan, because it possessed the tediously slow constricting faculty of a snake. He offered an offensive military design whereby there was to be a deep water blockade all down the eastern seaboard from Chesapeake Bay to the Florida Keys, then along the shore of the Gulf of Mexico to Matamoros. This would interfere with trade between the Confederacy and Europe, especially with the friendly British Isles whose hungry textile mills would gladly take southern cotton in exchange for whatever the Southerners desired—munitions, clothing, shoes, or other necessary goods. Then, according to Scott, he would send an army of 60,000 men, backed by gunboats, down the length of the Mississippi from Cairo, Illinois, past New Orleans. This would effectually cut off the South from the cattle and the grains of Texas and from anything else that might come from or through Mexico. When these moves had been accomplished the South would be forced to capitulate because of starvation and lack of military equipment. In this fashion, with trifling property damage and little bloodshed, the whole affair would be a relatively benign strife.

These, of course, were the ramblings of an old man, the thinking of one who as a colonel had fought the British on the Canadian border fifty years ago, and who as a flamboyant general had won a brilliant victory at Churubusco some fifteen years before. But such a warrior scarcely possessed the military competence or strategic vision demanded for this modern conflict. It was mandatory that the old soldier be put on the shelf.

True, the master design did have its defects. The navy was too small to blockade the entire coast; furthermore 60,000 men were insufficient to seize and maintain control of the Mississippi River. Even so, basically the idea had genuine merit. In the end the North won the war by destroying the ability of the South to fight. In essence this was accomplished along the lines the old general was trying to promulgate.

In the spring of 1861 the armchair tacticians and the politician strategists had the situation well in hand. There was no time for mere military planning. This was to be a short war and with a quick conclusion. "On to Richmond" was the battle cry, and nothing was to be gained by delay. There were, however, some unanticipated problems. Some of them were military, some were medical.

> In the early period of the war, the troops reached their destinations generally in a very unsatisfactory condition. . . . They were crowded into cattle cars as if they were beasts, frequently with empty haversacks, and with no provisions for their comfort on the road. Prompted by generous impulse, men and women boarded the trains as they halted at the stations in cities, and served the men hot coffee and such food as could most readily be provided. But it was only by accident, or through tireless and patient watching, that they were enabled to render this small service to their country's defenders: for no telegram announced the coming of the hungry men, not for long and weary months

was a system devised for the comfort and solace of the soldiers, as
they passed to and from the battle-field . . . Men stood for hours
in a broiling sun, or drenching rain, waiting for rations and
shelter, while their ignorant and inexperienced Commissaries
and Quartermasters were slowly and painfully learning the duties
of their positions. At last, utterly worn out and disgusted, they
reached their camps.

This was the situation in the Union army, but the soldiers
of the Confederacy were no better off. According to H. H.
Cunningham in *Doctors in Gray:*

The major cause of a large amount of sickness was the early
failure to prevent many who were unqualified for military service
from being inducted. Medical regulations prepared in 1861
directed surgeons to strip and examine recruits and screen out
those who were not physically and mentally fit, but . . . many
volunteers had been accepted who were ill-prepared to endure
the rigors of camp life. The volunteer system, asserted a leading
newspaper, "brings to the field the most patriotic, but the most
excitable and nervous portion of the population. These people,
however gallant in the field, have rarely the constitution to stand
the real burden of war."

And again we find the Medical Director of the Union
Army of the Potomac complaining, "It seemed as if the
army called out to defend the life of the nation had been
made use of as a grand eleemosynary institution for the
reception of the aged and infirm, the blind, the lame, and
the deaf, where they might be housed, fed, paid, clothed
and pensioned, and their townships relieved of the burden
of their support."

These were the armies that the North and the South
were mobilizing to fight the greatest struggle ever, up to
that time, to be engaged anywhere in the world.

Congress met in special session on July 4, 1861 and
authorized the President to recruit a half million men for
the duration of the war. Much against the advice of General Scott, who far more than any of the Union militarists
understood the spirit and potential of the South, Lincoln
allowed himself to be swayed by the persistent roar of "On
to Richmond." With no attempt at surprise—the newspa-

pers detailed every move, every rumor—General McDowell with his carefree, ill-trained, poorly equipped force crossed the Potomac on their way to make quick work of the capture of the Southern capital. On July 21 they met Beauregard's army near Manassas Junction behind a small stream known as Bull Run.

It was a very amateurish affray. On both sides the troops were poorly trained, their officers inexperienced. There was confusion regarding orders, flags and uniforms. For several hours the battle went this way and that. Suddenly Confederate reinforcements appeared, the Union lines began to fall back, the situation became impossible for the unskilled Union officers to handle and the retreat became a rout.

The politicians, the socialites, and the armchair strategists who had ridden out from Washington to witness the Confederacy being crushed in one swift blow frantically raced back, clogging rutted roads and narrow bridges, with one wide river to cross before reaching the capital. All next day and for days thereafter the completely disorganized Union forces straggled into the city. In his *History of the United States Sanitary Commission,* Charles J. Stillé wrote:

> The appearance of the streets was in the strongest possible contrast to that which could be imagined of a city placed by a strong necessity under the severe control of a military discipline. Groups of men wearing parts of military uniforms and some of them with muskets were indeed to be seen; but on second sight they did not appear to be soldiers. Rather they were a most woebegone rabble, which had perhaps clothed itself with the garments of dead soldiers left on a hard-fought battlefield. No two were dressed completely alike; some were without caps, others without coats, others without shoes. All were alike excessively dirty, unshaven, unkempt, and dank with dew. The groups were formed around fires made in the streets, of boards wrenched from citizens' fences. Some were still asleep, at full length in the gutters and on door steps, or sitting on the curbstones resting their heads against the lamp-posts. Others were evidently begging for food at housedoors. Some appeared ferocious, others only sick and dejected, all excessively weak, hungry and selfish. There was no apparent

organization; no officers were seen among them, seldom even a non-commissioned officer. At Willard's Hotel however, officers swarmed. They, too, were dirty and in ill-condition; but appeared indifferent, reckless, and shameless, rather than dejected and morose.

At this point the government itself, paralyzed and helpless, sent for General McClellan and charged him with the responsibility of reorganizing the army. It was a tough assignment. He had no intelligence service worthy of the name, although the rebels had informants everywhere in Washington. Also McClellan was a very competent, well educated, politically ambitious snob who had no admiration for Lincoln and no respect for the civilian administration. By November the drillmaster general had an aggregate of two hundred thousand men in the District and in Virginia but nobody moved. The bulletin that was telegraphed to the country each morning, "All quiet on the Potomac," became a standing joke. By December even the President was on the verge of despair and exclaiming, "What shall I do? The people are impatient; Chase has no money and he tells me he can raise no more; the General of the Army has typhoid fever. The bottom is out of the tub. What shall I do?"

For many months after Bull Run there was the most intense fear in Washington that the rebels might attack the utterly demoralized capital. There are some individuals now, over a century later, for whom it is still a mystery why such an attack, almost certain to succeed, never took place. The failure of such an advance was no mystery to the commander of the Confederate troops in the field, General Joseph E. Johnston. The numbers of sick in Johnston's army were literally staggering. On August 17 Johnston in camp at Manassas reported a total of 4,809 sick of 18,178 present, a ratio of greater than one in four. Much of the illness could be lumped under such categories as diarrhea and dysentery, and some of it could be diagnostically refined as typhoid fever. The causative factors were lack of latrines, lack of use of latrines, and improperly located latrines—they all combined to pollute the water and infect the food.

Nor was that summer's inactivity any mystery to General Robert E. Lee, in command of a sizeable force in the mountains of western Virginia, an area not yet separated from the seceding state. Lee hoped to retain the region for the Confederacy and also to strike northward. He failed in both attempts, and his own letters, many of them to his wife, eloquently tell the story of his travail.

Aug. 4, 1861. The soldiers everywhere are sick. The measles are prevalent throughout the whole army, & you know that disease leaves unpleasant results, attacks on the lungs, typhoid, &c., &c., especially in camp where accommodation for the sick is poor.

Aug. 9. The men are suffering from the measles, &c., as elsewhere . . .

Aug. 29. There has been much sickness among the men, measles, &c., & the weather has been unfavorable. . . . Although we may be too weak to break through their lines, I feel well satisfied that the enemy cannot at present reach Richmond. . . .

Sept. 1, 1861. We have a great deal of sickness among the soldiers, & now those on the sick list would form an army. The measles is still among them, though I hope it is dying out. But it is a disease which though light in childhood is severe in manhood, & prepares the system for other attacks. The constant cold rains, mud, &c., with no shelter but tents, have aggravated it. All these drawbacks, with impassable roads, have paralyzed our efforts. . . .

Sept. 3, 1861. Rain, rain, rain, there has been nothing but rain. . . . This state of weather has aggravated the sickness that has attacked the whole army, measles and typhoid fever. Some regiments have not over 250 for duty, some 300, 500, or about half, according to its strength. This makes a terrible hole in our effectives. . . .

Sept. 17, 1861. Our poor sick I know suffer much. They bring it on themselves by not doing what they are told. They are worse than children, for the latter can be forced.

There is no question that Lee was in desperate straits. In the late summer of 1861 he found himself stationed with an army of 17,000 in a supposedly healthful locality in the western Virginia mountains. Hardly had he encamped when the morning reports showed some 4,000 cases of disease with an extremely high rate of mortality. Soon investigation by the medical officer disclosed that the heavy rains were carrying the camp excreta directly into the sources of the water supply. Measles, of course, was another story. The Southern soldiers, far more than those from the Northern states, were country boys, many of whom had never been in contact with measles. This is a far more virulent ailment among adults than it is among children, and a century ago was indeed for all a more vicious disease than it is now. Under the cold, wet conditions of camp life with insufficient nutrition and inadequate medical care, the incidence of pneumonia and death and disability was far higher than would ever have been experienced otherwise. The armies of Joseph E. Johnston in northern Virginia in front of Washington and of Robert E. Lee in the western Virginia mountains in the final crucial months of 1861 were completely immobilized by disease. So we are faced with one of the many imponderables of history. Perhaps if the Confederates could have struck in the later months of 1861 . . . ? Is it possible that measles and typhoid fever determined the outcome of the war?

It was not until well after the New Year of 1862 that there was any significant military activity in the eastern theater. Then came the initial decision of the Federal high command. It was for an all-out frontal attack against Richmond. The Army of the Potomac under General McClellan was ordered to clash with the Army of Northern Virginia under the command of the awesome triumvirate of Generals Joseph E. Johnston, Jackson, and Lee.

McClellan was to rue the day, and the day was February 13, when he pontificated so sententiously, "In ten days I shall be in Richmond." He never did get there, although it was scarcely his fault. When Joe Johnston blocked his forward path by occupying Fredericksburg, Union plans were promptly altered to provide for a flanking attack. At the end of March the Navy transported the troops down the Potomac and around to the peninsula formed by the York and the James rivers, landing them below Yorktown. Here they found a nuisance confronting them. At Yorktown there was a garrison of 16,000 Confederate soldiers astride the path to Richmond. McClellan was properly disturbed at the thought of leaving such a force in his rear and across his supply line as he advanced up the peninsula. The trouble was he wasted far too much time, considering his vastly superior force, in dealing with the matter. His chief medical advisor, Dr. Charles S. Tripler, whose faults greatly outweighed his capabilities, nevertheless recognized as early as April 7 the hazards presented by a large swamp bordering the Union camps. Tripler astutely warned the general that the site was potentially malarious if the weather should turn warm, and that is what happened.

In a short time malaria and typhoid appeared. Aside from weakening the Federal forces the delay provided ample time for the Confederates to marshall their own defenses near Richmond. On May 4 Johnston secretly pulled his garrison out of Yorktown, having successfully held the large Union army at bay for an entire month, whereupon the Army of the Potomac proceeded to crawl through the mud on the York River side of the peninsula in the wake and through the typhoid-ridden campsites of the retreating rebels. It was a form of biological warfare, unrecognized and unintentional, but entirely real. By this time the main body of the Confederate army was now on the peninsula and prepared to contest each foot of soggy ground in defense of Richmond.

There was a sharp fight at Williamsburg, briefly delaying the advance, after which the Army of the Potomac slogged forward for two weeks until it was encamped in the swamps of the Chickahominy River less than a dozen miles from the Confederate capital. At this point two rations of whiskey and quinine were issued to the Union troops each day, and for years thereafter the very mention of the term "Chickahominy fever" would send a shudder through the survivors of that campaign.

Johnston's first real clash with McClellan took place at Fair Oaks on May 31 and ended in a draw, but Johnston himself was wounded and Lee assumed the command. During June there was much maneuvering over difficult, often submerged, terrain. This crucial month terminated with the Battles of the Seven Days, and both armies withdrew. Lee fell back into Richmond, which now became one vast hospital with every household tending its quota of sick and wounded. McClellan at the same time retired to Harrison's Landing on the James River where his exhausted men were based under the protection of the Navy's guns. Despite his losses, McClellan was by no means defeated, and he pleaded with Washington for reinforcements to carry on the attack against Richmond. He needed the reinforcements and Dr. Jonathan Letterman, his new medical director who had just succeeded the incompetent Dr. Tripler, tells us why.

> The troops for several consecutive days and nights had been marching and fighting among the swamps and streams which, abounding in this part of Virginia, render it almost a Serbonian bog. The malaria arising from these hotbeds of disease began to manifest its baneful effects on the health of the men when they reached Harrison's Landing. The labors of the troops had been excessive, the excitement intense; they were obliged to subsist on marching rations, and little time was afforded to prepare the meagre allowance. They seldom slept, and even when the opportunity offered, it was to lie in the mud with the expectation of being called to arms at any moment. . . . This marching and fighting in such a region, in such weather, with lack of food, want of rest, great excitement, and the depression necessarily consequent upon it, could have no other effect than that of greatly increasing the numbers of sick after the army reached Harrison's Landing. Scurvy existed in the army when it reached this point. The seeds had doubtless been planted by want of vegetables, exposure to cold and wet, working and sleeping in the mud and rain, and the inexperience of the troops in taking proper care of themselves under difficult circumstances. This disease is not to be dreaded merely for the numbers it sends upon the Reports of

Sick: the evil goes much further, and the causes which give rise
to it undermine the strength, depress the spirits, take away the
courage and elasticity of those who do not report themselves sick,
and who yet are not well. They do not feel sick, and yet their
energy, their powers of endurance, and their willingness to
undergo hardship, are in a great degree gone, and they know not
why.

Despite McClellan's pleas that with adequate troops
he could take Richmond that summer, the political powers
in the war department, terrified for their own safety,
ordered the army back to Washington to protect the city.
The Peninsular Campaign was ended at great cost in
casualties and lives on both sides, but Yankee feet would
not tramp the streets of Richmond for nearly three more
years.

Largely ignored, while the eastern theater of war was
aflame, was the vitally important conflagration in the west.
If the North was to cut off supplies to the Confederacy
from Louisiana, Texas, and Mexico it was essential that
the Union control the Mississippi River. The Ohio River,
which joins the Mississippi at Cairo, Illinois, is itself served
some fifty miles upstream from that juncture by the Tennessee and the Cumberland flowing northwest from Tennessee in a nearly parallel direction. Two earthworks, Fort
Henry on the Tennessee and Fort Donelson on the
Cumberland, closed these waterways to Federal traffic to
the interior. These then were key positions to the Confederate west, and capture of the two posts would open a
navigable waterway into the very heart of the western
Confederacy.

On February 6, 1862, after a sharp attack by Navy
gunboats, Fort Henry was reduced, and shortly thereafter,
again with naval help, and after a brisk overland march, an
unheralded officer named U. S. Grant demanded and received the "unconditional surrender" of Fort Donelson.
General Albert Sidney Johnston, based at Bowling Green,
was severely criticized for not sending strong reinforcements to Fort Donelson prior to the anticipated attack but

there is documentary evidence that widespread sickness in his own encampment made it impossible for Johnston to make such a move. In any case the failure was most significant. It meant that Nashville, potentially a large Confederate supply base, was to remain in Union hands for the duration of the war.

The next Federal military objective was Corinth, a small town in the northeast corner of Mississippi, important solely because it was a railroad junction. Generals A. S. Johnston and Beauregard had joined there for the defense of this valuable transportation center. The Southern commanders, determined that an offensive maneuver was the best defense, moved against Grant who was assembling his troops at Pittsburg Landing. With superior Southern forces they confidently expected to drive the Yankees into the Tennessee River. The fierce and bloody Battle of Shiloh was the result. There were huge losses on both sides. General Johnston bled to death from what should have been a nonfatal wound in the leg. Grant lost more men but held the field and Beauregard returned hastily to Corinth.

On April 11, General Halleck, unhappy about the publicity currently being showered on his subordinate U. S. Grant, took personal command of the Army of the Tennessee. After gathering a massive army of 100,000 men at Pittsburg Landing, Halleck managed to spend an entire month traveling the twenty-three miles to Corinth, entrenching every night on his ultra-cautious march. Historians comment that this gave Beauregard "plenty of time to withdraw the Confederate army intact" to Tupelo fifty-three miles farther south, but this is not exactly the way it was.

Beauregard in Corinth was surrounded by a ghastly scene. More than 5,000 wounded had been evacuated from the battlefield at Shiloh. Surgical care scarcely warranted the name. The tiny hospitals were soon overflowing with combat casualties. From the houses in the town, from porches, sidewalks, railroad platforms came the agonizing cries of the injured and the dying. But that was only a small part of the scene. In addition to the injured from the distant battlefield there were no fewer than 18,000 soldiers on the sick list feverish with malaria, dysentery, typhoid, and measles. Food and water were in short supply. Beauregard sent in his succinct report:

> The main purposes and end for which I occupied and held Corinth having been mainly accomplished by the last of May, and by the 25th of that month having ascertained definitely that the enemy had received large accessions to his already superior force, while ours had been reduced day by day by disease, resulting from bad water and inferior food, I felt clearly my duty to evacuate that position without delay.

The anxieties and dilemmas facing a commander in the field are not invariably appreciated at supreme headquarters. Jefferson Davis was profoundly disturbed at the decision to abandon this strategic position at Corinth and demanded to know more specifically why this retrograde action had been taken. Beauregard's reply was blunt:

> The retreat was not of choice but of necessity. The position had been held as long as prudence and the necessities of the case required. We had received our last available reinforcements. Our force was reduced by sickness and other causes to about 45,000 effective men of all arms. . . .

Two months earlier, when Grant had established his encampment at Pittsburg Landing it was then the consensus that the battle of Corinth would be the final conflict in the Confederate west. As it turned out, there was no battle of Corinth, and all that Halleck's Army of the Tennessee marched into was a deserted, gutted, smouldering ghost town where the ashes of Confederate equipment and supplies mingled with the ashes of Confederate dead.

Because of this hollow triumph, General Halleck was called to Washington and promoted to the command of all the Union armies. Halleck had never led, or directed, soldiers in combat, nor was he aware that Fortune's smile was a disdainful snicker. Flies, mosquitoes and microscopic agents had dealt his adversary a far more lethal blow than would ever have been delivered by Union soldiers and their ordnance.

In the campaign against "the Gibraltar of the Mississippi," as it is described by the general historians, Grant crossed to the west side of the river about twenty miles above the fortress, marched to about thirty miles below, and crossed back at Bruinsburg. He then fought his way north by a most circuitous route, and finally received the surrender on July 4, 1863. This was not the first campaign against Vicksburg. It was the fourth. Of the preceding three, two were medical reversals, and almost no one has ever heard of them.

In the spring of 1862 Federal rams and gunboats made quick work of the feeble fleet protecting Memphis, whereupon the river was clear for Union water traffic all the way south to Vicksburg. Late in April the navy's star performer, David Farragut, blasted his way up from the Gulf to receive the surrender of New Orleans, which was occupied a few days later by Major General Benjamin F. Butler. In another week Farragut was at Baton Rouge whereupon that town was taken over by Brigadier General Thomas Williams. The northward advance continued and the fleet with General Williams's troops aboard arrived at Vicksburg on May 18, 1862. The weather was steamy and hot and Williams took note:

> . . . the men have suffered from insufficiency of transportation, cramped and crowded more like live stock than men, without the means of exercise on board or room to form for inspection. Filth and dirt, with all the authority and supervision I could exert, abounded on vessels and men to a disgusting and of course most unwholesome degree. . . . the flooded country afforded no dry ground to land on. . . .

It soon became apparent that under these circumstances the defenses were far too strong so after a desultory engagement the vessels with their unwashed and sickly cargoes went downstream, the troops to Baton Rouge and the fleet to New Orleans.

In a few weeks both army and navy had been beefed up and by June 25 were in place for a second attack, only to discover that the Southerners had made the most of the delay to strengthen their defenses. By this time the spring flood waters had receded to allow one regiment to bivouac on the peninsula opposite the fortified town, but three others remained on board the transports. Malaria was soon prevalent. When the Seventh Vermont Regiment arrived on June 25 it counted 800 men fit for duty. Within three weeks more than 700 were on the sick list and there was no one to sound taps over the new graves. The Ninth Connecticut was no better off for the sick list was essentially the roll of the regiment and eventually 153 died. Naturally sickness was widespread in Vicksburg as well, but communication by land to the east was maintained, which meant that fresh troops and supplies could be poured in.

The last week in July, General Williams conceded defeat, and told one of the naval officers that of 3,200 men brought by him a month before there were only 800 fit for duty, the others were dead of disease or in hospital with fevers. Combat casualties had been negligible on both sides.

The third attempt against Vicksburg, the first from the land side, was launched in mid-winter so malaria was not a factor. This time the defenses were too strong and the swamps were too big. General Sherman had no choice but to retreat. The fourth attempt was the successful one in which Grant obtained the surrender of Vicksburg on the very day that Lee was retreating from Gettysburg. From the point of view of blood and glory and ordnance and oratory, Gettysburg was the turning point of the Civil War. From the military aspect Vicksburg was more important, because now the watery ring envisioned by Winfield Scott was closed around the Confederacy and the stage was being set for Sherman to march to the sea.

The medical history of the Civil War was by no means concluded in the summer of 1863, nor has the outline presented here been more than the briefest sketch of the significant events of the first two years. The available data is voluminous and the present attempt has been merely to describe certain situations in which disease appeared to be a decisive factor in the outcome of battles or campaigns that were fought, or in which the element of disease made combat impossible or so utterly impractical that it did not occur.

During the final two years of the war the armies on both sides were healthier than they had been previously. By then the soldiers were veterans, immune to many of the infectious ailments so prevalent earlier. Many organizational problems had been solved, particularly in regard to camp police, food supply, shelter, and clothing.

A most significant development for the North was the creation of the United States Sanitary Commission. This voluntary organization was established by a small group of dedicated individuals stirred by the horrors suffered by the British in the Crimea six years before. The Commission resolved to do for the Union soldiers what the administration in Washington and the army medical service were obviously unprepared to do. Opposition was strong—Lincoln scornfully referred to it as the fifth wheel to the coach—but political resistance faded under the growing impression that these people would do no harm.

Whatever lack of support the Sanitary Commission found in Washington was more than made up by the enthusiasm created back home where the soldiers came from. Millions of dollars were raised, great quantities of the comforts as well as the necessities of life were provided for the troops; transportation for the sick and wounded was arranged, surgical supplies were distributed, but most important of all, the Commission demanded and achieved vast improvements in camp sanitation.

There is no question that the organisms responsible for typhoid fever and dysentery, the virus of measles, and the malaria-bearing mosquitoes had no social or political motivations. The issues of secession or slavery bothered them not a whit. They attacked impartially, they disabled and killed impartially. Both sides were rendered inactive after the first Battle of Bull Run. In essence the same thing happened the following year after the fruitless campaign on the peninsula. The crucial victory of Vicksburg was delayed a full year because Union losses from disease could not be replaced as could those in the fortified town. Many other situations could be cited. There is but one conclusion that can be generally agreed on regarding the impact of disease on the outcome of the Civil War—it prolonged the conflict. There can be no doubt that time favored the North. Time exhausted the Confederacy whereas the North was militarily stronger in 1865 than it had been at any earlier date. In that sense disease was again decisive.

9

The Greatest Era

The Civil War was fought in the final moments of medicine's dark hour before the dawn. Countless thousands suffered miserably and many thousands died miserably because the candle of medical science was then unlit. In another decade the flame of that candle would flicker, in two decades it would burn dimly but steadily, and by the end of the century there would be a bright flame fed by new discoveries, new ideas, new tools. Then the flame itself would brighten to shed light on great expanding horizons. One of the great tragedies of the Civil War was that so much crippling and death among fighting men on both sides could have been avoided by the enlightenment soon to appear.

So frequently is the statement heard at the present time that there has been more progress made and more knowledge gained in the field of medicine in the past generation than in the previous two thousand years that we are in danger of believing our own propaganda and being convinced by our own clichés. There is an impressive list of achievements in our current era: antibiotics, anticoagulants, antihistamines, antihypertensives, oral substitutes for insulin in diabetes, chemotherapy for cancer, vaccines for a variety of illnesses such as influenza, poliomyelitis, measles, and mumps. In the hospitals there are now recovery rooms, intensive care units, cardiac monitors, radioactive isotopes, artificial kidneys, open heart and revascularization procedures, CAT (computerized axial tomograph) scanners, and organ transplants. Yet despite our present-day smugness all these "wonders of modern medicine" are only extensions of researches and techniques and extrapolations of ideas that germinated and flowered in Europe and America between 1865 and 1900.

On Saturday, October 1, 1870, a new scientific periodical, *The Medical Times,* made its initial appearance in Philadelphia. The leading article in the first issue was contributed by Dr. Samuel D. Gross, Professor of Surgery in the Jefferson Medical College, and one of the most distinguished surgeons in America. His paper dealt with the surgical management of strangulated hernia, and after a detailed discussion of the problem the renowned practitioner concluded that the treatment of choice for that life-threatening disorder was to pack it in ice.

Surgery was then in its most awkward age. Because of the abolition of pain during surgical procedures following the introduction of ether anesthesia in 1846, operations increased ten times in number, but unfortunately accompanying this innovation there were no corresponding advances in operative technique, in the management of wounds, or in the handling of the post-operative patient. "Civil surgery," J. Collins Warren of Boston later remarked, "came to have as high a mortality as that which marked the campaigns of the Napoleonic Wars." In the same vein Jonathan Mason Warren in his Annual Address to the Massachusetts Medical Society in 1864 commented somewhat ruefully that surgical wounds healed by first intention (that is without becoming infected) far more frequently a few miles out in the country than in the crowded and unhygienic Boston area. This was scarcely an original observation on the part of the elder Dr. Warren. Percival Pott had noted the same phenomenon a hundred years earlier in London. The concept that dirt, pollution, and crowded humanity were significant factors in surgical infection were slow to gain acceptance. In 1874 Sir John Erichsen, the professor of clinical surgery at University College Hospital in London, revealed the opalescence of his crystal ball when he pompously proclaimed, "the abdomen, the chest and the brain would be forever shut from the intrusion of the wise and humane surgeon."

Fortunately for ailing humanity there were already new ideas, new approaches, and new weapons against disease. Joseph Lister at the age of thirty-three had been appointed professor of surgery in the University of Glasgow. Among many others he had been pondering the problem presented by serious injuries occurring on Scottish farms and on Glasgow streets. He stated:

> The frequency of disastrous consequences in compound fracture, contrasted with the complete immunity from danger to life or limb in simple fracture, is one of the most striking as well as melancholy facts in surgical practice. If we inquire how it is that an external wound communicating with the seat of fracture leads to such grave results, we cannot but conclude that it is by inducing through access of the atmosphere, decomposition of the blood which is effused in greater or less amount around the fragments and among the interstices of the tissues, and, losing by putrefaction its natural bland character, and assuming the properties of an acrid irritant, occasions both local and general disturbance. . . . Turning now to the question how the atmosphere produces decomposition of organic substances, we find that a flood of light has been thrown upon this most important subject by the philosophic researches of M. Pasteur, who has demonstrated by thoroughly convincing evidence that it is not to its oxygen or to any of its gaseous constituents that the air owes this property, but to minute particles suspended in it, which are the germs of various low forms of life, long since revealed by the microscope, and regarded as merely accidental concomitants of putrescence, but now shown by Pasteur to be its essential cause, resolving the complex organic compounds into substances of simpler chemical constitution, just as the yeast-plant converts sugar into alcohol and carbonic acid.

Lister quickly grasped the significance of Pasteur's demonstration that there was no such thing as spontaneous generation. Germs did not spring out of nowhere. He then recalled the situation faced by the village fathers of Carlisle in the north of England where the residents were unhappy because of the odor of the local sewage disposal system. The town board discovered that the addition of carbolic acid to the sewage prevented putrefaction and eliminated the offensive odor. Lister recognized that this was a bacterial rather than a chemical effect and he then applied the carbolic acid approach to several cases of compound fracture and reported his results in the *Lancet* in 1867, and a new era in the history of surgery falteringly began.

"Falteringly" because Lister's ideas were by no means accepted with the alacrity that anesthesia had been welcomed. For one thing Pasteur's concepts were not universally well regarded. Much rethinking was required about long-established principles of wound healing and the laudability of pus. Perhaps most important, the Listerian method was not invariably successful. It failed partly because his technique was not properly emulated, but also because carbolic acid itself was sufficiently irritating to tissues so as to interfere oftentimes with wound healing.

Toward the end of the Franco-Prussian War both French and German surgeons began applying Lister's methods in military cases, where technique was readily adapted to field conditions. These doctors were sufficiently impressed with their results, compared to their previous experiences, that when they returned to civilian life they began searching for simpler methods to obtain the same beneficial effects. Neuber at Kiel boiled everything that might possibly come in contact with the operative site. From 1885 on he boiled dressings, bandages, instruments, overalls, and even the patients' clothing and the salt solution with which the wounds were irrigated. His results were excellent. Also in 1885 Ernst von Bergman and his assistant Schimmelbusch developed steam sterilizers, and the following year a French surgeon, Bedard, designed an autoclave and was the first to use steam under pressure to sterilize operating room supplies. By 1890 gowns were being used by Hayes Agnew in Philadelphia, and about the same time William S. Halsted in Baltimore began feeling sorry for his operating room nurse (whom he later married) who acquired a severe dermatitis on her hands from cleaning surgical instruments with mercuric chloride and car-bolic acid. He persuaded the Goodyear Rubber Company to make two pairs of thin rubber gloves for her to use. It was not until 1896, however, that Dr. Joseph C. Bloodgood, who had been Halsted's resident, began using gloves routinely in surgical operations. The rest of the operating room regalia gradually made an appearance. The cap was in use at least by 1904 by Halsted, but the face mask was not employed until some time later. It had taken an entire generation for the antiseptic era to give way to the age of asepsis, but the days when the surgeon whetted his knife on the sole of his shoe and wore a morning coat stiff with blood and pus to the amphitheater were fortunately fading memories.

In the meantime operative procedures were being de-veloped rapidly. By 1881, Billroth in Vienna had resected the esophagus and the pylorus of the stomach for cancer and had done a total laryngectomy. In 1886 Reginald Fitz of Boston solved an ancient problem when he published his classic paper on appendicitis, and three years later Charles McBurney at the Roosevelt Hospital in New York designated a point on the abdomen where pressure by the examining doctor gave indication that the appendix was inflamed. In 1892 Halsted read a paper entitled "The Radical Cure of Inguinal Hernia in the Male" in which he described a well-planned and anatomically sound curative approach. Thus in the space of twenty-two years a com-plete change in surgical thinking had occurred regarding one of the commoner afflictions of man. The ice pack of Dr. Gross was outdated forever, and the dreaded and often fatal abdominal pain of appendicitis was no longer the dire threat it had been.

In Bern, Switzerland, where goiters were endemic, Theodor Kocher directed his attention to the thyroid and in fifteen years had so perfected his technique that in 1898 he performed 600 thyroidectomies with only one death. Although we must assume that nearly all of these were colloid goiters, and hence much less likely to be accompanied by complications than overactive thyroid glands, the fact remains that another important surgical procedure had been standardized. So by now the basic principles of modern surgery had evolved. If one can control pain, hemorrhage, and infection, the horizons of surgery are enormously extended. The abdomen and the pelvis were now in the surgeon's realm. The central nervous system and the chest must wait for advances in basic physiology but the groundwork had been laid.

One instrument that was of inestimable value in the expansion of medical thought in the post–Civil War era was the introduction into clinical practice of the thermometer. It made its appearance in English hospitals about 1866 and was in general use in another four years. The original implements were clumsy and slow to register and were about ten inches long. Readings were usually axillary. Within a short time Sir Clifford Allbutt aided in the origin of the pocket thermometer. In 1868 Carl Wunderlich of Leipzig wrote his masterpiece on the relationship of animal heat to health and disease. He stated:

> There are two well-ascertained facts, which not only justify us in endeavoring to determine the temperature of the body in diseases, and render the use of the thermometer both a duty and a valuable aid to diagnosis, but form the basis of all our investigations. The first fact is the *constancy of temperature in healthy persons,* or, in other words, that healthy human beings of every age and condition, in all places and in all circumstances, and exposed to all kinds of influences, provided these do not impair health, have an almost identical temperature. The second fact is the *variation of temperature in disease,* for in sick persons we are constantly meeting with deviations from the normal temperature of the healthy.

The meticulous study that followed demonstrated conclusively that fever was a symptom of many disorders and not a disease in itself. This concept, which seems so obvious now, represented a real departure from established doctrines dating back a thousand years.

The stethoscope, in one form or another, had been in use since 1819, enabling the examining physician to understand much of the workings of the heart and the lungs. The next instrument of any value in measuring the function of the circulatory system did not appear for sixty years, and even then was only a research toy. This was the first accurate implement for the estimation of the blood pressure without requiring an arterial puncture, and was devised by von Basch in 1880. His method consisted of obliterating the arterial pulse by means of a ball filled with water and measuring the pressure within the ball at the moment the pulsations disappeared. Potain improved the instrument by using a ball half filled with air attached to an aneroid manometer. In 1896 Riva-Rocci at the Italian Congress of Medicine demonstrated a new apparatus for the estimation of the blood pressure. This consisted of a rubber bag surrounded by a cuff of inelastic material and connected with a mercury manometer and a rubber bulb. Essentially it is the instrument in use today.

No matter how commonplace and even trivial the introduction of the fever thermometer and the blood pressure machine may seem in the late twentieth century they are still two of the basic instruments used to monitor the course of disease in every hospital in every civilized nation in the world. They were products of the era we are now discussing.

The modern student of medical history is frequently baffled by what appeared to be, in ancient times, a relative lack of interest in the heart. The intestinal tract, the spleen, and the lungs were considered important, but the organ that received the greatest attention was the liver. During the final third of the nineteenth century, however, the situation showed signs of change. The value of nitroglycerin as a means of relief for angina pectoris was announced in the *Lancet* in 1879. Of considerably more importance was an obscure contribution of a little known physician of St. Louis, Dr. Adam Hammer. Back in 1848 Dr. Hammer had taken part in the revolution in Germany then in progress. Inasmuch as he turned out to be on the losing side in this particular conflict, he chose to emigrate to St. Louis where he practiced surgery. In a Viennese periodical he published in 1878 a description of two individuals whose occlusion of the coronary arteries he had diagnosed during life and confirmed at autopsy. Incidentally, the third instance of death due to obstruction of the coronary arteries from atheromatous degeneration to be reported in America was in November 1883 and the heart was that of the foremost gynecologist of his era, Dr. J. Marion Sims.

At the end of the Civil War, surgery, except for the employment of ether and chloroform anesthesia, had advanced little since medieval times. At the end of the century, appendectomies, gall bladder removals, and bowel resections were routine procedures, at least in the academic community, and Halsted had published the definitive operation for the radical removal of cancer of the breast. Medical progress, at the same time, was demonstrated by the development of the clinical thermometer and the blood pressure machine, but to a much greater extent by the birth and growth of the science of bacteriology.

The concepts announced by Pasteur were now about to mature. Following the discovery of the spirillum of relapsing fever in 1873, advances in microbiology literally came tumbling after each other. In the next decade the amoebae causing one important form of dysentery were found: the fact, already suspected by Lister, that traumatic infections were due to bacteria was proven, and the gonococcus, the staphylococcus, the streptococcus, the typhoid bacillus, the malarial parasite, the tubercle bacillus, and the bacilli responsible for glanders in horses and diphtheria in children were all isolated. Before the end of the century the organisms responsible for cholera, tetanus, Malta fever, and plague were known, and the meningococcus had been pinpointed. Now, not only the causative organisms of many infectious diseases had been largely revealed, their means of attack were at last becoming understood.

Etiologic enlightenment was not the only progress

made during these years. Vaccination by means of attenuated, that is, weakened, organisms was announced by
Pasteur in 1880. The following year in the dramatic and
convincing experiment in the farmyard at Pouilly le Fort,
he demonstrated that sheep could be successfully immu-
nized against anthrax, an absolute scourge in France. A
landmark in microbiology and in preventive medicine had
been achieved.

A further advance was the finding that certain bacteria
killed their victims not by direct invasion and multiplica-
tion but by establishing a locus of activity, such as in the
throat, or in a contaminated wound, and from there sending out a poison—a toxin—which was carried by the blood-
stream while the germs remained at the point of entrance.
In this fashion the toxin fatally damaged distant tissues
such as cells in the heart muscle or in the central nervous
system. Two such common organisms were diphtheria and
tetanus bacilli. By 1890 von Behring had produced diphtheria antitoxin on an experimental basis and shortly
thereafter it was being used clinically. Although its acceptance was slow, it was ultimately recognized that when
properly used early in the infection the favorable results
were startling.

The most complex, confused, illogical branch of therapeutics since ancient times has been that of pharmacology—the use of drugs in medicine. A German practitioner,
Samuel Hahnemann, early in the nineteenth century had
made an attempt to bring some sort of order out of pharmaceutical chaos by relating the action of a given drug to
the symptoms of disease it appeared to mimic. He established the cult of homeopathy that survived for nearly a
century, but the basic premises under which it functioned
were so grossly in error that its contributions to scientific
knowledge were trifling.

Basically, in early days, there were two types of
medication: those employing metallic salts of mercury,
lead, arsenic, antimony, etc.; and the botanicals, substances derived from plants. The latter comprised the major-

ity of the medicinals in use prior to 1870. There had been certain very valuable discoveries early in the nineteenth century, namely that plants owe their poisonous as well as their medicinal properties to small quantities of active principles present in their leaves, stems, flowers or roots and are susceptible to chemical extraction and isolation. These facts demonstrated that certain substances could be administered in pure form and by the isolation of a few potent alkaloids, nitrogenous substances ordinarily of vegetable origin that form salts with acids and are usually obtained from dicotyledonous plants. From the discovery of alkaloids came several valuable drugs such as morphine, strychnine, cocaine, atropine and especially quinine.

There was another group of chemical substances isolated in the early years of the nineteenth century, namely the glycosides. These are generally crystalline solids soluble in water. The first of this group to be isolated was salicin, obtained from willows in an impure state in 1825, and in a pure form in 1829. It is the active principle of the very ancient remedy for rheumatism, oil of wintergreen. Salicylic acid was introduced into internal medicine in 1874 when a process was developed for producing it synthetically on a commercial scale. This was a genuine turning point. Pharmaceutical manufacturing was no longer a matter merely of processing plants. Drugs could be produced in the test tube and another new world of medical thought and imagination opened up.

In a very sketchy fashion this discussion has dealt with the changes in thought and approach that developed in the ancient modalities of medicine and surgery in the latter third of the nineteenth century. Now we must turn our attention to a generic idea that even its discoverer had not dreamed of prior to the moment it appeared in his vision. In 1895, at Würzburg, while working with a vacuum tube, William Conrad Roentgen accidentally found that shadows were formed on a photographic plate. On December 28, 1895 he read a paper before the Würzburg Society, the first two paragraphs of which were as follows:

If the discharge of a fairly large induction-coil be made to pass through a Hittorf vacuum-tube, or through a Lenard tube, a Crookes' tube, or other similar apparatus, which has been sufficiently exhausted, the tube being covered with thin, black cardboard which fits it with tolerable closeness, and if the whole apparatus be placed in a completely darkened room, there is observed at each discharge a bright illumination of a paper screen covered with barium platinocyanide, placed in the vicinity of the induction-coil, the fluorescence thus produced being entirely independent of the fact whether the coated or the plain surface is turned toward the discharge-tube. This fluorescence is visible even when the paper screen is at a distance of two meters from the apparatus. It is easy to prove that the cause of the fluorescence proceeds from the discharge-apparatus, and not from any other point in the conducting circuit.

There is nothing to be gained by quoting further from this historic document with its ponderous Teutonic grammar. It is fascinating, considering the extent of foot-dragging by surgeons in accepting the basics of antisepsis and asepsis, and the dilatory tactics of medical men in grasping the importance of the newer therapeutics, to observe the alacrity with which the medical profession immediately clutched to its bosom the discovery of Dr. Roentgen. Although a few New England Puritans protested that the privacy of clothed womanhood would be invaded, the essential idea was promptly put to use throughout the civilized world.

Before the next year was out Dr. Francis Henry Williams at the Boston City Hospital published a classic account in the *Boston Medical and Surgical Journal* dealing with the use of the fluorescope [sic] in the examination of the chest. His comments eight decades later are still poignant:

The picture which presents itself to the eye when the body is examined by the fluorescope is full of interest. The trunk appears lighter above than below the diaphragm and the rise and fall of the muscle are distinctly seen; the chest is divided vertically by an ill-defined dark band which includes the backbone; and each side is crossed by the dark outline of the ribs, the spaces between which, are the brightest portion of the picture. One also sees the pulsating heart, especially the ventricles, and under favorable conditions the right auricle and left auricle, but it is difficult to separate the latter from the pulmonary artery; a small portion of one side of the arch of the aorta may be seen in the first intercostal space to the left of the sternum. The organs of the abdomen are much less readily observed, but the presence of a piece of lead or of substances impermeable to the Roentgen rays may be detected in them. The neck and face may be reached with the fluorescope; and in the arms and legs the bones and certain foreign substances may be seen. The head is the least promising field.

The advantages provided by X-ray films in military surgery were promptly and conclusively demonstrated by the Medical Department of the United States Army during the Spanish-American War. Fractures were visualized and bullets and shrapnel located in the extremities, chest, and skull. In 1898 a medical student at Harvard, Walter B. Cannon, used bismuth as a contrast medium to study the physiology of digestion in the goose and another technique in diagnostic radiology became available.

It would appear from the foregoing that the final third of the nineteenth century was a period of continuous progress in medical science, and in many respects that is true. There was to be, however, one vigorous and lethal backlash perhaps to remind mankind that it was still too soon to assume that supremacy over Nature was at hand. Again the theater was war.

The Spanish-American War is not a source of great national pride. It might not have happened at all except for the ambition and avarice of Mr. William Randolph Hearst of the *New York Journal* and Mr. Joseph Pulitzer of the *New York World,* and their hyperactive hirelings. The newspapers sponsored and covered the war and determined for all time the military reputations of Theodore Roosevelt and Leonard Wood. The Rough Riders galloped off into history mounted on frothing chargers, but they climbed San Juan Hill on shank's mare.

It was a weird war. In March 1898 Congress appropriated $50,000,000 for national defense and placed it at the disposal of President McKinley. Of this, the Medical Department, which was forbidden by law to accumulate reserve supplies in peacetime, was allotted $20,000 to squander as it might. This bounteous financial preparation was for a campaign in which typhoid fever in the training camps and tropical diseases in the field would kill more than fourteen times as many men as enemy action.

Despite what is remembered about the affair now, the Santiago campaign was not under the direction of a pair of personable individuals named Roosevelt and Wood. There was a commanding general who resented the fact that when he sailed from Tampa in the heat of June he had with him seventy-one medical officers and eighty-nine newspaper correspondents along with his 17,000 troops. The general was William Rufus Shafter and he had the dubious distinction of being the largest general officer who ever commanded an American army in the field; he weighed 310 pounds. Despite his bulk he was a capable commander. His fat was not between his ears. His error was that he made no attempt to butter up the fourth estate. For their part, the correspondents buried him under an avalanche of news despatches glorifying the two colorful colonels and to this day Shafter has never been exhumed.

He succeeded in driving the enemy back from the landing area but soon found himself in an extremely uncomfortable spot. The Spanish were entrenched high on a hill in the city of Santiago. The enemy had the advantage of terrain, there were formidable barbed wire defenses, and the Spaniards outnumbered the Americans. But the most ominous threat was from attack—the yellow fever season was at hand.

Shafter had several alternatives. He could retreat, because he still had his beachhead and naval superiority. He could hurl his forces against the Spanish stronghold, but a fortified city is seldom subjected to frontal attack except by superior strength either in troops or in firepower, or at least without the element of surprise. Shafter had none of these. He could lay siege to the city and starve the enemy, but he knew that yellow fever would do more harm to his men than to his acclimated opponent. There was one other alternative that would only have occurred to an American. In the face of overwhelming odds and with time running out, Shafter demanded the surrender of the Spanish—and got it.

The capitulation occurred on July 17, less than a month after the landing, and it was none too soon. Malaria and yellow fever abruptly reduced the victorious army to such a shambles that it had to abandon Cuba in a hurry and withdraw to ill-prepared cantonments rapidly thrown up on desolate stretches of Montauk Point.

Yellow fever succeeded in driving most of the combat troops of the American army from Cuba, but it was a temporary triumph and a final major victory. Two years later the Medical Department delivered the disease a fatal blow when its Yellow Fever Commission headed by Dr. Walter Reed proved beyond doubt that its vector was the *Aedes aegypti* mosquito. Although the isolation of the specific virus was not accomplished for several years, the organism was powerless without a mode of transportation, so control of the disease was at hand.

This is the story of one-third of a century in the history of medicine. In 1865 surgery, except for the highly important discovery of general anesthesia, was as primitive as it had been for two thousand years. Medicine had survived an orgy of excessive bleeding and purging, but was still only capable of treating symptoms. Public health was a matter of quarantine, a concept dating back to the fifteenth century. Radiology was not even a dream in the imagination of the most learned minds of the generation. Yet in the brief time that it took for the nineteenth century to turn into the twentieth, modern surgery sprang into being, febrile disease was separated into entities, drug therapy began to make sense—and progress—and radiology was born and almost immediately achieved adolescence. Surely this was medicine's greatest era.

Bibliography

Adams, George Worthington. *Doctors in Blue*. New York: Henry Schuman, 1952.

Adams, Henry. *History of the United States of America*. 9 vols. New York: Charles Scribner's Sons, 1891–1896. Reprint. New York: Antiquarian Press, 1962.

Allen, Gardner W. *A Naval History of the American Revolution*. 2 vols. Boston: Houghton Mifflin, 1913.

Allison, R. S. *Sea Diseases*. London: John Bale, 1913.

Andrist, Ralph K. *The Long Death: The Last Days of the Plains Indians*. New York: Macmillan, 1964.

Ashburn, P. M. *A History of the Medical Department of the United States Army*. Boston: Houghton Mifflin, 1929.

———. 1947. *The Ranks of Death*. New York: Coward-McCann.

Augustin, George. *History of Yellow Fever*. New Orleans: Published by the Author, 1909.

Balfour, Andrew and Scott, Henry Howard. *Health Problems of the Empire*. New York: Henry Holt, 1924.

Bancroft, George. *History of the Colonization of the United States*. 10 vols. Boston: Little, Brown, 1872.

Bancroft, Hubert Howe. *History of California*. 2 vols. San Francisco: A. L. Bancroft, vol. 1, 1884, vol. 2, 1886.

———. 1884. *History of the Pacific States—The Northwest Coast*. vol. 2. San Francisco: A. L. Bancroft.

Baurmeister, Carl Leopold von. *Revolution in America*. Translated and annotated by Bernhard A. Uhlendorf. New Brunswick: Rutgers University Press, 1957.

Belcher, Henry. *The First American Civil War*. vol 1. London: Macmillan, 1911.

Bernheim, Bertram M. *The Story of the Johns Hopkins*. New York: Whittlesey House, 1948.

Bigelow, Jacob. *American Medical Botany*. 3 vols. Boston: Cummings and Hilliard, 1817.

———. 1867. *Modern Inquiries*. Boston: Little, Brown.

Blake, John B. *Benjamin Waterhouse and the Introduction of Vaccination*. Philadelphia: University of Pennsylvania Press, 1957.

Blanton, Wyndam B. *Medicine in Virginia in the 17th Century*. Richmond: William Byrd, 1930.

————. 1931. *Medicine in Virginia in the 18th Century.* Richmond: Garrett & Massie.

————. 1933. *Medicine in Virginia in the 19th Century.* Richmond: Garrett & Massie.

Borden, W. C. *The Use of the Roentgen Ray by the Medical Department of the United States Army.* Washington: Government Printing Office, 1900.

Boyd, Mark F. "An Historical Sketch of the Prevalence of Malaria in North America." *American Journal of Tropical Medicine* 21 (March 1941).

Bridenbaugh, Carl. *Cities in the Wilderness.* New York: Capricorn, 1964.

Buchan, William. *Domestic Medicine,* 3rd American ed. Boston: John Trumbull, 1778.

Buley, R. Carlyle. *The Old Northwest.* 2 vols. Bloomington: Indiana University Press, 1951.

Burpee, Lawrence J. *The Discovery of Canada.* Toronto: Macmillan, 1938.

Calder, Isabel M. ed. *Colonial Captivities, Marches and Journeys.* New York: Macmillan, 1935.

Carter, Henry Rose. *Yellow Fever.* Baltimore: Williams and Wilkins, 1931.

Catton, Bruce. *A Stillness at Appomattox.* New York: Doubleday & Co., 1954.

————. 1956. *This Hallowed Ground.* New York: Doubleday & Co.

Cendrars, Blaise. Translated from French by H. L. Stuart. *Sutter's Gold.* New York: Harper & Bros., 1926.

Chambers, J. S. *The Conquest of Cholera.* New York: Macmillan, 1938.

Chardon's Journal at Fort Clark. Abel, Annie Heloise, ed. Pierre: Fox, 1932.

Chisholm, C. *Malignant Pestilential Fever.* London: C. Dilly, 1795.

Churchill, Edward D. ed. *To Work in the Vineyard of Surgery: The Reminiscences of J. Collins Warren.* Cambridge: Harvard University Press, 1958.

Clinton, Sir Henry. *The American Rebellion.* Edited by Willcox, William B. New Haven: Yale University Press, 1954.

Creighton, Charles. *A History of Epidemics in Britain.* 2 vols. Cambridge: Cambridge University Press, 1891.

Cunningham, H. H. *Doctors in Gray.* 2nd ed. Baton Rouge: Louisiana State University Press, 1960.

Cushing, Harvey. *The Life of Sir William Osler.* 2 vols. Oxford: Oxford University Press, 1925.

DeVoto, Bernard. *Across the Wide Missouri.* Boston: Houghton Mifflin, 1947.

————. 1952. *The Course of Empire.* Boston: Houghton Mifflin.

————. 1963. ed. *The Journals of Lewis and Clark.* Boston: Houghton Mifflin.

Diaz del Castillo, Bernal. *The Discovery and Conquest of Mexico.* Translated by A. P. Maudslay. New York: Farrar, Straus and Cudahy, 1956.

Dick, Everett. *The Sod-House Frontier.* New York: D. Appleton-Century, 1937.

Donnan, Elizabeth. *Documents Illustrative of the History of the Slave Trade to America.* 4 vols. Washington: Carnegie Institution, 1932.

Dow, George Francis. *Slave Ships and Slaving.* Salem: Marine Research Society, 1927.

Dowdey, Clifford and Manarin, Louis H. *The Wartime Papers of R. E. Lee.* New York: Bramhall House, 1961.

Drake, Daniel. *Principle Diseases of the Interior Valley of North America.* 2 vols.: vol. 1 Cincinnati: W. B. Smith, 1850; vol. 2 Philadelphia: Lippincott, Grambo, 1854.

Drury, Clifford M. *Marcus Whitman, M.D.* Caldwell: Caxton Printers, 1937.

Dubos, René and Jean. *The White Plague.* Boston: Little, Brown, 1952.

Duffy, John. *Epidemics in Colonial America.* Baton Rouge: Louisiana State University Press, 1953.

Duncan, Louis C. *Medical Men in the American Revolution.* Carlisle Barracks: Medical Field Service School, 1931.

Flexner, Simon and Flexner, James Thomas. *William Henry Welch and the Heroic Age of American Medicine.* New York: Viking, 1941.

Flint, Austin. *Clinical Medicine.* Philadelphia: Henry C. Lea, 1879.

Foreman, Grant. *Advancing the Frontier.* Norman: University of Oklahoma Press, 1933.

————. 1932. *Indian Removal.* Norman: University of Oklahoma Press.

Fortescue, J. W. *A History of the British Army.* 13 vols. London: Macmillan, 1899–1930.

Freeman, Douglas Southall. *George Washington: A Biography.* 7 vols. New York: Charles Scribner's Sons, 1948.

Gallup, Joseph A. *Epidemic Disease in the State of Vermont.* Boston: T. B. Wait & Sons, 1815.

Garrison, Fielding H. *An Introduction to the History of Medicine.* 3rd ed. Philadelphia: W. B. Saunders, 1924.

Gibson, James E. *Dr. Bodo Otto and the Medical Background of the American Revolution.* Springfield: Charles C. Thomas, 1937.

Gipson, Lawrence Henry. *The Great War for the Empire.* New York: Knopf, vol. 7, 1949: vol. 8, 1953.

Gordon, Maurice Bear. *Aesculapius Comes to the Colonies.* Ventnor, N.J.: Ventnor Publishing Co., 1949.

Graham, Harvey. *The Story of Surgery.* New York: Doubleday, Doran, 1939.

Graves, Rt. Hon. Thomas Lord. *The Graves Papers.* Edited by F. E. Chadwick. New York: Naval History Society, 1916.

Gross, S. D. "On the treatment of strangulated hernia." *Medical Times.*
    1 (Oct. 1, 1870).

Hahnemann, Samuel. *Organon of the Art of Healing.* Translated by C.
    Wesselhoeft. 5th American ed. New York: Boericke & Tafel, 1883.

Hamilton, Charles ed. *Braddock's Defeat.* Norman: University of Okla-
    homa Press, 1959.

Hamilton, Peter J. *Colonial Mobile.* Boston: Houghton Mifflin, 1897.

Handlin, Oscar. *The Uprooted.* New York: Grosset & Dunlap, 1951.

Hart, Francis Russell. *Admirals of the Caribbean.* Boston: Houghton
    Mifflin, 1935.

————. 1929. *The Disaster of Darien.* Boston: Houghton Mifflin.

Heagerty, John J. *Four Centuries of Medical History in Canada.*
    Toronto: Macmillan, 1928.

Hirsch, August. *Handbook of Geographical and Historical Pathology.*
    Edited by Charles Creighton. 3 vols. London: New Sydenham
    Society, 1883.

Holmes, Oliver Wendell, "The Contagiousness of Puerperal Fever."
    New England Quarterly Journal of Medicine 1, 1843.

Hosmer, James K. *History of the Louisiana Purchase.* New York:
    Appleton, 1902.

Howarth, David. *The Golden Isthmus.* London: Collins, 1966.

Hrdlicka, Ales. "Disease, Medicine and Surgery Among the American
    Aborigines." *Journal of the American Medical Association.* 99
    (Nov. 12, 1932).

————. 1908. *Physiological and Medical Observations among the In-
    dians.* Washington: Government Printing Office.

————. 1909. *Tuberculosis Among Certain Indian Tribes of the
    United States.* Washington: Government Printing Office.

Hutchinson, Thomas. *The History of the Colony and Province of
    Massachusetts Bay.* Edited by Lawrence Shaw Mayo. 3 vols. Cam-
    bridge: Harvard University Press, 1936.

James, W. M. *The British Navy in Adversity.* London: Longmans,
    Green, 1926.

Johnson, Allen and Corwin, Edward S. *The Age of Jefferson and
    Marshall.* New Haven: Yale University Press, 1921.

Johnston, Henry P. *The Yorktown Campaign.* New York: Harper &
    Bros., 1881.

Keevil, J. J. *Medicine and the Navy.* vol 1. Edinburgh: E. & S. Living-
    stone, 1957.

Kelly, Howard A. and Burrage, Walter L. *American Medical Biog-
    raphies.* Baltimore: Norman, Remington Co., 1920.

Kenton, Edna ed. *Jesuit Relations and Allied Documents.* New York:
    Albert and Charles Boni, 1925.

Kraus, Michael. *The United States to 1865.* Ann Arbor: University of
    Michigan Press, 1959.

Larsell, O. *The Doctor in Oregon.* Portland: Oregon Historical Society,
    1947.

Leech, Margaret. *Reveille in Washington*. New York: Harper & Bros., 1941.

Letterman, J. *Medical Recollections of the Army of the Potomac*. New York: Appleton, 1866.

Lind, James. *A Treatise on the Scurvy*. 2nd ed. London: A. Millar, 1757.

Lister, Joseph. "On A New Method of Treating Compound Fracture." *The Lancet* 1 (1867). Reprinted in *Medical Classics*. vol 2. Baltimore: Williams and Wilkins, 1937–38.

Livermore, Mary A. *My Story of the War*. Hartford: A. D. Worthington, 1889.

Livermore, Thomas L. *Numbers and Losses in the Civil War*. Bloomington: Indiana University Press, 1967.

Lounsberry, Alice. *Sir William Phips*. New York: Charles Scribner's Sons, 1941.

MacKenzie, Alexander. *Voyages from Montreal Through the Continent of North America*. 2 vols. New York: New Amsterdam, 1902.

Mahan, A. T. *The Influence of Sea Power Upon History*. Boston: Little, Brown, 1918.

Major, Ralph H. "The History of Taking the Blood Pressure." *Annals of Medical History*, New Series: vol. 2 (January, 1930).

Major, Robert C. "Aboriginal American Medicine, North of Mexico." *Annals of Medical History*, New Series vol. 10 (November, 1938).

Mann, James. *Medical Sketches of the Campaigns of 1812, 13, 14*. Dedham: H. Mann & Co., 1816.

Marryat, Frederick. *A Diary in America*. New York: Knopf, 1962.

Mather, Cotton. *The Diary of Cotton Mather*. Boston: Collections of Massachusetts Historical Society, 1911–1912.

Mathews, John Joseph. *The Osages*. Norman: The University of Oklahoma Press, 1961.

Maxwell, William Quentin. *Lincoln's Fifth Wheel*. New York: Longmans, Green, 1956.

Medical and Surgical History of the War of the Rebellion. vol. 1, part 3. Edited by Charles Smart. Washington: Government Printing Office, 1888.

Millis, Walter. *The Martial Spirit*. Cambridge: Literary Guild, 1931.

Minter, J. E. *The Chagres, River of Westward Passage*. New York: Rinehart, 1948.

Morison, Samuel Eliot. *John Paul Jones: A Sailor's Biography*. Boston: Little, Brown, 1959.

———. 1952. *Of Plymouth Plantation*. New York: Knopf.

———. 1965. *Oxford History of the American People*. New York: Oxford University Press.

Myer, Jesse S. *Life and Letters of Dr. William Beaumont*. St. Louis: C. V. Mosby, 1939.

Olmsted, Frederick Law. *A Journey in the Seaboard Slave States*. New York: G. P. Putnam's Sons, 1904.

Osler, William. *Practice of Medicine.* New York: D. Appleton & Co., 1892.

Packard, Francis R. *The History of Medicine in the United States.* Philadelphia: J. B. Lippincott, 1901.

Parkman, Francis. *The Works of Francis Parkman.* Frontenac Ed. 16 vols. New York: Charles Scribner's Sons, 1915.

Partridge, B. *Sir Billy Howe.* New York: Longmans, Green, 1932.

Patterson, A. Temple. *The Other Armada.* Manchester: The University Press, 1960.

Phillips, Paul C. *Medicine in the Making of Montana.* Missoula: Montana State University Press, 1962.

Pickard, Madge E. and Buley, R. Carlyle. *The Midwest Pioneer: His Ills, Cures, and Doctors.* New York: Henry Schuman, 1946.

Pringle, John. *Observations on Diseases of the Army.* 2nd ed. London: Millar, Wilson and Durham, 1753.

Quaife, Milo M. *Chicago and the Old Northwest.* Chicago: University of Chicago Press, 1913.

Reed, William Howell. *Hospital Life in the Army of the Potomac.* Boston: William V. Spencer, 1866.

Riedesel, Major General. *Memoirs and Letters and Journals During His Residence in America.* 2 vols. Translated by William L. Stone. Albany: J. Munsell, 1868.

Riedesel, Mrs. General. *Letters and Journals Relating to the War of the American Revolution.* Translated by William L. Stone. Albany: J. Munsell, 1867.

Roberts, Kenneth. *March to Quebec.* New York: Doubleday & Co., 1953.

Roberts, W. Adolphe. *The French in the West Indies.* Indianapolis: Bobbs-Merrill, 1942.

Roentgen, William Conrad. "On a New Kind of Rays" (1895). *Source Book of Medical History.* New York: Dover, 1960.

Rose, J. H. *Life of Napoleon.* 2 vols. London: G. Bell & Son, 1913.

Rosenberg, Charles E. *The Cholera Years.* Chicago: The University of Chicago Press, 1962.

Rowse, A. L. *The Elizabethans and America.* New York: Harper & Bros., 1959.

Sappington, John. *The Theory and Treatment of Fevers.* Arrow Rock: Published by the Author, 1844.

Scott, Leslie M. "Indian Diseases as Aids to Pacific Northwest Settlement." *Oregon Historical Quarterly,* 29 (1928).

Singer, Charles and Underwood, E. Ashworth. *A Short History of Medicine.* 2nd ed. Oxford: Clarendon Press, 1962.

Smillie, Wilson G. *Preventive Medicine and Public Health.* New York: Macmillan, 1947.

————. 1955. *Public Health: Its Promise for the Future.* New York: Macmillan.

Snively, William D. Jr. and Furbee, Louanna. "Discoverer of the Cause of Milk Sickness." *Journal of the American Medical Association.* 196 (June 20, 1966).

Sparks, Jared. *The Writings of George Washington.* Boston: J. B. Russell, 1834–37.

Stearn, E. Wagner and Stearn, Allen E. *The Effect of Smallpox on the Destiny of the Amerindian.* Boston: Bruce Humphries, 1945.

Steiner, Paul E. *Disease in the Civil War.* Springfield: Charles C. Thomas, 1968.

————. 1968. *Medical-Military Portraits of Union and Confederate Generals.* Philadelphia: Whitmore.

Stillé, Charles J. *History of the United States Sanitary Commission.* Philadelphia: J. B. Lippincott, 1866.

Strong, Richard P. *Diagnosis, Prevention and Treatment of Tropical Diseases.* 6th ed. 2 vols. Philadelphia: Blakiston, 1943.

Tarleton, Lt. Col. *History of the Campaigns of 1780 and 1781 in the Southern Provinces of North America.* London: T. Cadell, 1787.

Thacher, James. *A Military Journal.* 2nd ed. Boston: Cottons and Barnard, 1827.

Thomson, Samuel. *A Narrative of the Life and Medical Discoveries of Samuel Thomson.* Boston: Printed for the Author by E. G. House, 1822.

Trease, George Edward. *Pharmacy in History.* London: Balliere, Tindall and Cox, 1964.

Trevelyan, Sir George Otto. *The American Revolution.* 6 vols. New York: Longmans, Green, 1908.

Tucker, Glenn. *Poltroons and Patriots.* 2 vols. Indianapolis: Bobbs-Merrill, 1954.

Vallery-Radot, René. *The Life of Pasteur.* Translated by Mrs. R. L. Devonshire. New York: Doubleday, Page & Co., 1923.

Ward, Christopher. *The War of the Revolution.* 2 vols. New York: Macmillan, 1952.

Waring, Joseph Ioor. *A History of Medicine in South Carolina.* Columbia: South Carolina Medical Association, 1964.

Warshaw, Leon J. *Malaria: The Biography of a Killer.* New York: Rinehart, 1949.

Whitlock, Brand. *La Fayette.* 2 vols. New York: D. Appleton & Co., 1929.

Willcox, William B. "The British Road to Yorktown: A Study in Divided Command." *American Historical Review* 52 (Oct., 1946).

Williams, Francis H. "A Method for More Fully Determining the Outline of the Heart by Means of the Fluorescope Together with Other Uses of This Instrument in Medicine." *Boston Medical and Surgical Journal* 135 (1896).

Williams, Herbert U. "The Epidemic of the Indians of New England 1616–1620." *Johns Hopkins Hospital Bulletin* 20 (1909).

Williams, Samuel Cole ed. *Adair's History of the American Indians.* New York: Argonaut, 1966.

Winslow, Charles-Edward Amory. *The Conquest of Epidemic Disease*.
    Princeton: Princeton University Press, 1944.
————. 1952. *Man and Epidemics*. Princeton: Princeton University
    Press.
Winsor, Justin ed. *Narrative and Critical History of America*. 8 vols.
    Boston: Houghton Mifflin, 1889.
Wrong, George Mackinnon. *Conquest of New France*. New Haven:
    Yale University Press, 1918.
Wunderlich, Carl Reinhold August. "Body Temperature in Health and
    Disease (1868)." Reprinted in *Source Book of Medical History*.
    New York: Dover, 1960.
Zinsser, Hans. *Rats, Lice and History*. Boston: Little, Brown, 1935.

Index

Indians (*cont.*)
  in Canada, 11, 12, 30
  cholera among, 40–41
  in colonial America, 5–8, 10, 14,
    17–18, 26–31
  French and Indian War and, 86,
    91, 92
  malaria among, 36–38
  measles among, 39–40
  of the Northwest, 35–41
  Queen Anne's War and, 74
  smallpox among, 5–8, 30–34
  tuberculosis among, 41
  venereal disease among, 35–36
  see also individual tribes
Influenza, 173
Iroquois, 4, 5, 11
  King William's War and, 64–66
  Queene Anne's War and, 75–76
Isle aux Noix, 100

Jackson, Robert, 118, 122–23, 136
Jamaica, 158, 161
James, Robert, 88, 89
Jenkins, Robert, 52
Jenkin's Ear, War of, 52–57
Jenner, Edward, 176
Jesuit Relations and Allied Documents (Kenton, ed.), 4
Johnson, Sir William, 90
Johnston, Albert Sidney, 204
Johnston, Joseph E., 199, 201

Kalm, Peter, 30
Kemble, Stephen, 59–60, 62
Kentucky, 169–70
Keppel, Augustus, 143
King William's War, 64–74
Kiowa, 40
Kocher, Theodor, 215

Lafayette, Marquis de, 131, 138–42,
  147–48
LaJonquiere, Rear Admiral, 85
Las Casas, Bartolomé de, 2
Leclerc, Charles Victor Emmanuel,
  165–67
Lee, Robert E., 200, 203
Leprosy, 27
Leslie, General, 125, 129, 136
Letterman, Jonathan, 203
Lettsom, John C., 176
Lewis, Meriwether, 31–32, 35–36

Lincoln, Abraham, 195, 197, 199
Lind, James, 153–55
Lister, Joseph, 213–14
Livingston, Robert, 68, 69
Longueuil, 86
Louisbourg, 77
  War of the Austrian Succession
    and, 78–82, 85
  French and Indian War and, 86,
    93
Louisiana, 150, 153, 154, 163, 167
Louisiana Purchase, 149
Louis XIV, king of France, 64–66
Lovell, Joseph, 107–8

McBurney, Charles, 215
McClellan, George, 199, 201–4
MacKenzie, Alexander, 31
Madison, James, 102
Maine, colonial, 66
Maitland, General, 163
Malaria (ague; intermittent fever),
  18, 62, 86, 151, 162, 170, 186
  in Africa, 25
  during American Revolution,
    112–13, 122–23, 132–36
  during Civil War, 202, 203, 208
  in Florida, 155, 158
  among Indians, 36–38
  quinine for treatment of, 189
  in Spanish-American War, 224
  during War of 1812, 108
Mandans, 33–34
Mann, James, 107–9
Marryat, Frederick, 169–70
Martinique, 151, 163
Maryland, colonial, 18
Massachusetts, American Revolution
  and, 96
Massachusetts Bay Colony, 66–68
Massasoit, 6
Mather, Cotton, 72–74
Mather, Increase, 7
Measles, 39–40
  during Civil War, 200, 201
Medical Times, 212
Michigan, 170
Micmacs, 84
Milk-sickness (trembles), 190–93
Minnetarees, 34
Mississippi River and valley, 154–56,
  164
Mobile, 154, 155, 158